D0811973

Springer Series on ADULTHOOD and AGING

Volume 1 **Adult Day Care** Philip G. Weiler et al. O.P.

Volume 2 **Counseling Elders and Their Families:**
Practical Techniques for Applied Gerontology
John J. Herr and John H. Weakland

Volume 3 **Becoming Old:** An Introduction to Social Gerontology
John C. Morgan

Volume 4 **The Projective Assessment of Aging Method (PAAM)**
Bernard D. Starr, Marcella Bakur Weiner, and Marilyn Rabetz

Volume 5 **Ethnicity and Aging**
Donald E. Gelfand and Alfred J. Kutzik, with 25 contributors

Volume 6 **Gerontology Instruction in Higher Education**
David A. Peterson and Christopher R. Bolton O.P.

Volume 7 **Nontraditional Therapy and Counseling with the Aging** S. Stansfeld Sargent et al.

Volume 8 **The Aging Network:** Programs and Services, 2nd ed.
Donald E. Gelfand

Volume 9 **Old Age on the New Scene**
Robert Kastenbaum, with 29 contributors

Volume 10 **Controversial Issues in Gerontology**
Harold J. Wershow, with 36 contributors

Volume 11 **Open Care for the Aging:**
Comparative International Approaches
Virginia C. Little

Volume 12 **The Older Person as a Mental Health Worker**
Rosemary McCaslin, with 11 contributors

Volume 13 **The Elderly in Rural Society:** Every Fourth Elder
Raymond T. Coward and Gary R. Lee, with 16 contributors

Volume 14 **Social Support Networks and the Care of the Elderly:** Theory, Research, and Practice
William J. Sauer and Raymond T. Coward, with 17 contributors

Volume 15 **A Basic Guide to Working with Elders**
Michael J. Salamon

Michael J. Salamon, Ph.D., involved in the field of aging and adult development for over ten years, has worked in both community and institutional settings as a social service worker, administrator, clinician, researcher, and educator. He has published extensively on issues related to gerontology and geriatrics. Through the Adult Developmental Center, a private organization Dr. Salamon helped establish, he has been a consultant to a variety of professional groups in the United States and abroad. He has also served as professional advisor to a number of radio and television shows and is book review editor for *Clinical Gerontologist*. Dr. Salamon is presently a Clinical Supervisor at the New Hope Guild Community Mental Health Center in Brooklyn, New York.

A BASIC GUIDE TO WORKING WITH ELDERS

Michael J. Salamon, Ph.D.

SPRINGER PUBLISHING COMPANY
New York

Springer Publishing Company, Inc.
536 Broadway
New York, NY 10012

86 87 88 89 90 / 5 4 3 2 1

Library of Congress Cataloging-in-Publication Data

Salamon, Michael J.
Basic practices in applied gerontology.

(Springer series on adulthood and aging ; 16)
Bibliography: p.
Includes index.
1. Social work with the aged—United States. 2. Aged—Care and hygiene—United States. 3. Aged—Medical care—United States. 4. Aged—United States—Recreation. I. Title. II. Series.
HV1461.S24 1986 362.6'042'0973 86-965
ISBN 0-8261-5190-6

Printed in the United States of America

Contents

Acknowledgments

Authoring a book is often described as a long and arduous task. Despite the many intense hours invested over the course of several years, the difficult task of preparing this work became a highly rewarding one. Beginning with Dr. Max Pollack, who was the first professor to cajole me subtly into recognizing my interest in the field of gerontology, to my present colleague and regular collaborator, Dr. Vincent Conte, who always challenges me to try harder, I have received both the moral and pragmatic support necessary to following through on the completion of this text. I also must give thanks to the patients, residents, tenants, and participants of facilities and programs for the aged, as well as the administrators and clinical care staff, both in the United States and abroad. They were always encouraging, responded positively to suggestions, and never hesitated in taking part in the evaluation and applied research that, of necessity, was performed. I would like to list all of them, but that would be a formidable task. I therefore must thank them as a group.

A special debt of thanks goes to my typists, Maria Vicinanza and Linda Borzesi, for their punctuality as well as true interest; to my editors Barbara Watkins and Dr. Bernard Starr for their very constructive comments and suggestions; and most of all to Naomi, my wife, who did all of this and more. She typed, edited, cajoled, empathized, made suggestions, took a personal interest, promised it would be done on time and delivered, and kept the door to the study closed.

Preface

Over recent years it has become evident that there is a shortage of professionals trained to deal with the needs of the ever increasing number of aged people. This professional shortage is not unexpected, nor is it inexplicable. It is only within the last four decades that we have begun to witness the explosive growth of the percentage of elderly persons surviving well into their eighties. This growth has brought with it an increasing need for health, psychological, and social care.

While we have known bits of information regarding the aging process for many years, we have not had a sufficiently broad data base from which to prepare a science of aging. This dearth of information has caused the development of myths, biases, and stereotypes against working with the elderly as a group, and even against the aged themselves. Recently many of the myths and biases have been debunked, and now more individuals view entering the fields of geriatrics and gerontology as a worthy professional challenge. In fact, gerontology has been targeted as a growth field in a time of overall shrinking in the need for professional health care. Still, data are sparse and those that exist are not well unified. Little wonder then, that now, as we begin preparing greater numbers of students to work with the aged, we still have questions regarding what are the most appropriate methods of health care and the best emotional and social support systems.

Scientific investigators continue to make great strides in understanding the aging process. Research findings generally have limited merit unless they are ultimately put to use where they are most needed. This does not mean devising cures for the aging process; no one has yet stumbled upon the fountain of youth. What it does mean is that we explore better ways to provide health care, social stimulation, mental orientation, and emotional support to a group of individuals with unique needs, and translate those findings to the applied setting.

This text is based upon several years of lectures given in universities, hospitals, and nursing homes, to a variety of different professionals, all interested in gaining a better understanding of the field of gerontology and the needs of the aged. The lectures, while based on contemporary scientific information, were geared toward the provision of care. This text therefore is designed as a guidebook for service providers and students in the field of gerontology, whether or not these individuals are trained gerontologists and geriatricians. This book consolidates the most current information on the provision of care to the aged, with little of the work devoted to theory or philosophy.

The main body of the book consists of eight chapters. The first three provide a general overview of the field of applied gerontology. Chapter 1 is a review of human service programs, both formal and informal, and how they operate. The second chapter details the variety of health care services and the range of health care options available to older adults. The mental health needs of older adults are detailed in Chapter 3. The remaining five chapters of the text move from theoretical emphasis and overview to focus in more detail on practical issues. Chapter 4 provides information on community needs assessment techniques and outreach. The next chapter is a primer of interview techniques for the elderly in general, as well as those with special needs. Chapters 6 and 7 provide a detailed plan for the organization of recreation and socialization activities from both an administrative and management aspect, as well as giving specific suggestions for types of activities to use in organizing groups and resources. The final chapter explores techniques for the evaluation of program effectiveness. It is hoped that this book will provide useful guidelines for the provision of services, suggest useful techniques, and orient workers to the special needs of this age group.

No distinction is made by age in this text, as, for example, between the young-old and the old-old. In the provision of care in a community center, clinic, or nursing home, these distinctions are rarely made; therefore, in this text the terms *aged*, *elderly*, and *older adult* are used interchangeably. Similarly, little distinction is made between who provides what service. In an applied setting it is not uncommon for a registered nurse to perform tasks often performed by a social worker or recreator, or for a social worker to act as an advocate or program administrator.

It is my hope that this book will challenge the reader to reach a better understanding of the aging process, the needs of the aged, and how best to respond to these needs.

A BASIC GUIDE TO WORKING WITH ELDERS

1

How Human Service Programs Work

All of us have heard or read of dramatic situations in which older adults have needed the assistance of organized (usually public) care and service providers. The "bag lady" suffering from malnutrition and hypothermia and living in the darkest corners of big-city parks and railway stations could receive the protective services often offered by General Social Services, a government-funded organization. The services would include hospitalization, shelter, food, and possibly counseling. The media also have made familiar to us the disheartening situation of isolated elders living in constant fear of crime. They often live in apartments with no utilities, and although it is available, they often do not know how to get assistance.

While these cases occur with more frequency than are tolerable, they are by far not the most common types of situations for which older adults need assistance. Only a small proportion of older adults are in need of long-term institutional care, yet almost all older adults, at least once in their later years, will become known to a social- or human-service provider.

DEFINITIONS

It is best to define our terms at this point, to make it clear what services are and who might offer them. A *social-service provider* or *human-service provider* is any individual who provides for the social, emotional, and/or physical needs of a client. These providers may have had formal training in a professional field such as medicine, nursing, psychology, social work, or public health; or they may simply be interested individuals with no specific professional training but with a special sensitivity.

The services provided may include counseling, information and referral, direction on how to apply for government entitlements, and advocacy for special needs. The issues involved in these services include, but are certainly not limited to, arranging for special housing needs, planning recreation activities; giving directions on where and how to get the appropriate types of health care; explaining the proper use of medications; and planning for wills, estates, and the resolving of other legal issues.

Over 80 percent of older adults have at least one chronic medical condition (Allan & Brotman, 1981). Included in these are arthritis, hypertension, heart conditions, hearing and visual impairments, and diabetes. Despite needing a moderate amount of medical supervision, however, most older people are capable of carrying on their daily routines. In addition to health care needs, most older individuals, including an increasing number of women (Kalish, 1975), have retired from work. On the average, an older retired person will live 20 years past retirement (Streib, 1971; Verbrugge, 1983), and how to use their remaining years is a primary issue. The transition from working to not working can be difficult, but it becomes even more difficult when related problems arise. These problems include decreased income, having to find new friends or social supports, and simply learning how to spend one's newly found free time. If not properly handled, these changes can cause a depressive illness to arise. This makes it clear why a broad range of services is needed.

This chapter will first discuss common social needs and circumstances of older adults and then explore the range of presently available programs that can help maintain or improve elders' quality of life. There are currently few service organizations that offer a complete range of social and human services. Most provider organizations offer a limited variety of service programs designed to meet certain needs. No distinction will be made as to whether programs are governmentally funded or are supported by private institutions. Except in cases where government entitlements are discussed, little is gained by making the distinction as to the source of funds. The range and depth of need suggest the importance of funding from as many sources as possible.

COMMUNITY DWELLERS AND THEIR SUPPORT GROUPS

In this section we will look at the sources of social interaction and support available to elderly community residents, that is, individuals who live in their own home or apartment. These individuals are similar to people of any age in that our lives are often defined by the company we keep. Our friends, our workmates, the religious groups we participate in, where we live, and who we live with all contribute to the person we are. To the degree that we gain a sense of identity from those with whom we interact, we are said to be part of a social group. Our social circle provides us with many of the supports we need for our well-being.

Informal supports are those resources that an individual has available through relationships with individuals or groups within the community. These supports are provided to older adults in their own homes and make them feel more secure. Informal caregivers provide emotional support and also are involved in an exchange of goods and services. These networks cannot provide the full range of necessary services, but they are the most responsive and adaptable of all of the support networks (Carp, 1976). These relationships take place on a variety of levels and usually follow a culturally dictated method of interaction.

Family support is also very important. The closest relationships among people tend to be with family members, in particular, with spouses or children. While family members tend to live nearby their older relative, however, they are not the only source of social contact and support. *Friends and neighbors* fill the vast majority of social support needs for older adult community residents.

The Marital Dyad

For most married people of all ages, their spouse is their primary source of social and emotional support. Many studies indicate that having a supportive marital partner helps people to overcome a number of stressful life circumstances (Cobb & Kasi, 1977; Gore, 1978). Some studies suggest that a positive, albeit slight, association exists between being married and reporting a higher level of life satisfaction (Edwards & Klemmack, 1973; Spreitzer & Snyder, 1974). Other researchers have found that if a male spouse is ill or incapacitated, his healthy wife will report a lowering of her own level of well-being, so intertwined is the marital relationship (Fengler & Goodrich, 1979). (This occurs whether the wife provides the direct care or not.)

There are some individuals who do not have the luxury of a spouse for sharing, social support, and reciprocity of care. The practice of men marrying women who are younger than themselves, combined with the generally lower life expectancy for men, results in a greater proportion of single women in the population. The overwhelming majority, almost 85 percent, of those whose spouses have died are women (Metropolitan Life, 1977). In the United States, widowhood occurs at about age 56 (U.S. Department of Commerce, 1980). By age 75, as many as 70 percent of American women are widowed. For men, the figure is closer to 29 percent. The death of a spouse is an extremely trying time for the surviving spouse. Aside from profound feelings of sorrow, anxiety, and even guilt (Peterson, 1979), an entire series of social relationships is radically changed. Relationships built on the common interests and friendships of the couple no longer exist (Butler & Lewis, 1976). Other family members are often turned to for the support they may provide in these instances; however, these supports may not truly fulfill the need (Monk, 1979).

Families

Families, however, do in fact provide one of the best forms of all-around informal support. Older adults often turn to their middle-aged children for assistance with many of their needs. The popular stereotype of older adults abandoned by their children is a myth (Brody, 1978). Contacts with adult children are frequent for older Americans; in fact, a large proportion, fully 73 percent, live within 30 minutes' traveling time of one another. This includes the 18 percent of those over 65 who live in the same household with one of their children (Cantor, 1981; Hays, 1984). The most frequently cited source of help for an older person, according to a 1982 U.S. General Accounting Office survey, is the older adult's child. Most often, it is a daughter assisting an aged mother (Sweetster, 1964). Studies further suggest that over 50 percent of home help services an older adult receives is provided by family and friends. The services provided include assisting with personal care, tidying up the home or apartment, preparing and serving meals, shopping, banking and other daily living activities.

While the family is a major form of support for the older American, there are times when the needs of an older parent or grandparent may become too taxing for family members. In fact, government programs are often structured in such a way as to encourage the family to remain less involved in the care of their older adult relative. In particular, Medicare and Medicaid are designed to provide assistance to older adults only if they are institutionalized, not if they are cared for at home. Further, while families are instrumental not only in assisting their older adult in getting to a health care provider but also in caring for a good many of their needs, a pilot study suggests that family members' understanding of the older adult's needs is not always consistent with that of the older adult (Rakowski & Hickey, 1981). This might suggest that older adults prefer not to burden their family support network, and so they hide many of their real needs. If this is true, it indicates an inadequacy in family support that needs to be remedied in some way.

Surveillance

Elderly apartment and home dwellers keep in touch with their community and neighbors in a variety of different ways. Perhaps the most basic is by looking out at the world from windows or porches. The outside space that is seen from within the individual's dwelling is known as the *surveillance zone.* Rowles (1981) has said that "the surveillance zone represents a primary focus of participation in the world beyond the threshold" of one's own home (p. 310). Sitting on one's porch or at the window may seem like a passive act, but it is an important component in community contact and participation. Not only does one watch activities that go on beyond the home, but one watches out for the normal events to happen. Should they not take place, the watcher is alerted. If Jenny, who normally sits on her porch, doesn't see Laura across the street open her window shades at 10 A.M., Jenny will call to see if Laura has a problem. Patterns of watching develop, and neighbors watch out for and are in turn watched by one another. Rowles has suggested that as active physical involvement decreases—for instance, when one retires and begins to spend more time at home—the passive involvement offered by a community surveillance zone increases.

Balanced Reciprocity

In the case of neighbor watching out for neighbor, the sheer act of reciprocity insures that the relationship will continue, but there are other subtle exchanges that go on to insure that the network will remain strong and committed. *Balanced reciprocity* (Sahlins, 1965), or the exchange of equivalent goods or services, is basic to the maintenance of the informal helping network. The type of exchange and how rapidly it takes place help to determine the nature of the relationship. There are two types: immediate exchange and deferred exchange.

Exchanges that take place immediately and are of an equivalent value to the service provided indicate the desire on the part of the recipient to keep the obligation to a minimum; hence, the relationship remains a limited one. Exchanges of this nature usually take place between individuals who may be considered friends but are not close. Myrtle needs to get to her doctor. None of those people close to her who normally would assist her with transportation are available, so she decides to call an acquaintance, Sarah, from down the block. Myrtle asks Sarah for help and offers to pay her for the cost of the ride. Sarah consents to take her.

If Sarah accepts the monetary reimbursement, that will signal that the relationship should remain a distant one. Sarah, however, tells Myrtle, "Don't be so foolish," and she refuses to accept the exchange. Deferring the act of exchange indicates a sense of trust; in doing this, Sarah has signaled a willingness to make the relationship a closer one. Myrtle understands the act of kindness, and she, in exchange, invites Sarah, who was recently widowed, over for dinner a few nights later. Both have signaled that they are willing to exchange services on a deferred and hence more involved level. It is reasonable to believe that this hypothetical relationship can develop into a strong and caring one (Wentowski, 1981).

One means of guaranteeing security in informal social-support relationships in old age is through *long-term reciprocity*, that is, taking part in balanced exchanges over long periods of time. A type of "credit" is built up so that when one is in need, there is a legitimate right to seek assistance, to "spend" some of the credit. Parents who have provided for the needs of children have this type of credit reserve. When the older adult parent is in need they can feel a legitimate right to seek assistance from their offspring. Spouses rely on each other in the most basic form of reciprocity relationships. If, however, the older adult is unmarried and childless, who is there to turn to? A recent study (Johnson & Catalano, 1981) indicates that, in cases like these, older adults turn for assistance to individuals whom they have accumulated as social resources over many years. These include kin, most often in the form of nieces and nephews, and close contacts who have been friends for many years.

Regarding reciprocity, the question often arises as to whether it is proper for a human-service professional to accept gifts, particularly when the relationship is a therapeutic or counseling one. The professional should always remember to keep the relationship on the appropriate level. It occasionally is appropriate for small gifts to be accepted, as these tokens of appreciation may encourage the relationship to proceed more effectively. If it becomes clear, however, that the intent of the gift is to develop a long-lasting dependency, then it must be made gently but firmly clear to the client that the nature of the involvement is professional.

Political Groups

The elderly are a heterogeneous group, sometimes conceived of as consisting of young-old (ages 60–74) and old-old (age 75 and over) (Neugarten, 1974). Yet, Rose (1965) suggests that older adults in America are beginning to form one large, cohesive social group. He found that there is an identification between older Americans because of their common concern with the issues affecting them. As a result, older individuals are beginning to turn to one another for help in dealing with their problems. In turn, they are, requesting responses to their needs by becoming politically active and lobbying for programs. Some proof for this comes from the fact that older adults vote more frequently than other adults and in general have higher levels of interest in the political process (Brotman, 1977; Glenn & Grimes, 1968; Jones, 1977). There is also the possibility that older adults join political groups simply for the camaraderie. Political action groups, regardless of the reason one joins them, may be seen as one form of social support.

The Work Environment

For those older adults still involved in work, the primary source of social interaction comes from the work setting. This social interaction with co-workers is one of the best forms of social support. The major portion of workers' waking hours are spent with individuals with whom they share a work environment. Not only does the environment provide workers with a center for social relationships, it also provides individuals with a regulated lifestyle, requiring that they be at work between given hours on specified days. It also provides for a sense of accomplishment through the reward of income, and it affords a full range of meaningful experiences. Work has even been referred to as a "jumping off point for interaction with the world" (Friedman & Havighurst, 1954).

There have been changes in this century that have undercut this area of support. Over 65 percent of the males in America aged 65 and over were actively involved in the labor force at the start of the twentieth century. By 1980, however, only 20 percent of this same group remained active in the workforce. There are projections that suggest that, by 1990, the figure will be about 15 percent. On the other hand, participation by older adult women in the workforce has remained relatively stable over the past 80 years. In 1900, just under 10 percent of women aged 65 and older worked full time, and it is estimated that by 1990 the figure may drop to just under 8 percent (U.S. Senate Special Committee on Aging, 1982).

It is clear that only a small proportion of older adult workers have the social supports of their work setting to call upon in times of need. While there are equivocal data as to whether retirement has a generally negative impact on the physical and mental health of older adults (Kasl & Berkman, 1981), there is little doubt that the adjustment—away from the general supports of the work setting and the social support it offers, to other avenues of social interaction—can be trying (O'Meara, 1977).

Voluntary Associations

There are other social ties which older adults may use to provide themselves with the social supports they need. These include voluntary associations such as clubs and religious organizations. To use but one example, active involvement in senior citizen center activities is a positive predictor of self-reported well-being, as well as of overall higher levels of satisfaction with life (Toseland & Sykes, 1977). These results may be somewhat tempered by other factors, in particular, health and socioeconomic levels: Healthier, wealthier people find it easier to get around (Ward, 1979). There is little doubt that the more involved older adults are, the happier they report themselves to be. The reverse also appears to be true: Individuals who report not having enough friends or who find themselves poorly integrated into their primary social network tend to report more illness and use health care services more frequently (Shuval, Antonovsky, & Davies, 1970).

Religious Organizations. Churches, temples, synagogues, and other religious organizations comprise an informal support system so important to people that the Committee on Family and Community Support Services of the White House Conference on Aging has formally suggested it be incorporated into the continuum of support services (White House Conference on Aging, 1981). These organizations have long played a major role in the lives of older Americans. The religious sector has begun to provide a growing number of services to older people in a wide variety of areas, in addition to counseling. These include recreation, fellowship, transportation, health care, home visiting services, nutritional programs, and housing assistance. Some studies have suggested that as individuals age their frequency of church attendance declines, despite increases in religious feelings (Moberg, 1968). More recently, however, surveys indicate that older Americans attend church regularly. Most older adults report having a religious preference, and many religious organizations report that fully 25 percent of their membership is over the age of 65 (The Gallup Report, 1982).

Senior Citizen Clubs. Often older adults will join together to formalize their social support network. Card groups, mah-jong players, golf partners, or even handball partners may join with each other on a regularly scheduled basis. These meetings are not simply for the sport but include the pleasures of company and caring interaction. Other groups include dancers, political action groups, church and temple related groups, health groups, and even self-help networks. The one overriding aspect of a seniors' club is the fact that it has been organized and run by older adults, for older adults. All members of the club have defined roles in the organization and are expected to follow through on their obligations to the group. In exchange, the group will react to members' needs, within the organizational charter of the group. The organizational charter need not be a formal document, and in the case of clubs it often is not. It is, however, an agreed-upon mode of interaction among group members.

Clubs fulfill a major purpose in the lives of their participants; however, they tend to have a limited membership. Membership may not be exclusionary by direction. A self-selection process, however, does tend to favor healthier people and those who are better off financially. They are the ones who have the resources to attend regularly and pay whatever fees, monetary or otherwise, the group may require for its continuation. Fees may be modest, for example, a nickel a pot for card players, or preparing a salad for a luncheon get-together. But the fees are an integral part of the reciprocity interaction. Furthermore, the payment of fees suggests to the participants that a commitment to the club has been made (Salamon, 1981) making it a more valued activity.

Individuals who, for example, regularly share park benches are not considered to be partners in a clublike organization. It is important to make this distinction. Unless there is an exchange in the form of a valued interaction, it makes little difference who one sits next to on the bench. One individual will not call on the other to provide social support beyond mere passing interaction. If, on the other hand, the individuals choose to meet at the same location on a regular basis and begin an ongoing interaction, they have begun a partnership that may build into a strong form of informal support. Most clubs begin this modestly. Spouses tend to come along, and park frequenters will stop by to comment on the chess moves the players make, or they may challenge the winner. As the weather grows inclement, what has become a regular series of games, complete with interested onlookers, moves to an indoor location and the group relationship is on its way to becoming cemented.

Senior citizen clubs can form anywhere older adults gather on an informal basis. Reasons for the formation of clubs are limited only by the interests of the members of the group. Clubs fulfill a number of goals for the participants:

- The participant is made to feel part of a caring network.
- All participants are active in that their sheer presence at organizational meetings makes them part of the groups interactions.
- They receive assistance and comfort from other group members and have found the social supports necessary to overcome loneliness and isolation.

The Senior Citizen Center. On occasion, informal senior citizen clubs grow so large that the group members decide to seek the assistance of someone, perhaps an outsider, to act as an administrator. When a club becomes formal both in terms of administrative structure and bringing in outside funding, then the club becomes a center.

These voluntary center programs had their start in the 1940s. In 1947, the Philadelphia Center for Older People and the San Francisco Senior Centers first opened their doors. Both of these programs were funded by the private voluntary sector and are considered to be among the first senior citizen centers in the United States. By the mid 1950s, most states had a number of senior centers. By 1959, the first state association of senior citizen centers was formed in Ohio. The association was to act as an overseer and advisor to the various funded centers in Ohio. In 1965, Congress passed the Older Americans Act, which provided funds for a variety of programs that would meet the needs of the elderly in America. The programs were to be administered by the newly formed Administration on Aging. In the act, senior citizen centers were identified as a major tool for the delivery of services to the elderly. One year later, in 1965, the National Council on Aging, a private voluntary organization devoted to expanding knowledge regarding aging, published its first directory of senior centers, which at that time numbered 360. Four years after that, in 1969, the National

Council on Aging established the National Institute of Senior Centers (NISC), which published the second national directory of senior centers in that year. By then, the list included 1,200 centers. By 1981, over 8,000 senior citizen centers were listed (NCOA, 1981).

The term *senior citizen center* can describe a variety of different places serving a range of people. Generally the participants of senior citizen centers are ambulatory, can get around on their own, and are of average physical and emotional health. Centers provide a variety of activities and services to older adults in both individual and group settings. These programs may be offered directly by the center or by groups wishing to reach older adults in places where they are known to congregate. Senior centers have been referred to as community focal points for services to the elderly (Jacobs, 1980).

Centers originally were designed as places where older adults could receive their service needs with dignity, thus enhancing their continued involvement in the community. For example, in 1972, Title VII of the Older Americans Act established a federally funded program to provide congregate meals to older adults. Today, about one-third of all the congregate meal sites are currently in senior centers; therefore, in addition to responding to the recreational and socialization needs of the elderly, senior centers have taken on an active role in maintaining the nutritional needs of the participants.

Federal funding for senior citizen centers, which has increased dramatically since the passage of the Older Americans Act in 1965, is channeled from the federal government through an Area Office on Aging or a State Office on Aging. It is the responsibility of these organizations to assess the needs of the older adults being serviced. These organizations have the further responsibility of supervising the centers in specified catchment areas. In some states or in areas where there are many centers, there may be a local Area Office on Aging serving a more direct supervisory function.

While there is no such place as an "average" senior center, it is not inappropriate to attempt to generalize the daily activities in a "typical" senior citizens center. Our typical center opens its doors at 8:30 in the morning and is open Monday through Friday, all year round. The staff of the center consists of a director, bookkeeper/secretary, cook, and possibly an assistant director who, along with the director, is also responsible for scheduling programs and providing direct social services to center participants. The assistant director complements the role of director by expanding the capability of service provision. In this typical center there are weekly program activity sheets posted at the main entrance. The listing includes activities such as bingo, dance, a variety of discussion groups on topics as varied as current events and consumer activism, and a variety of arts and crafts activities. Also scheduled is a health-education group. Some of the activities are run internally by the director, the assistant director, or one of the elderly participants who is a volunteer. The more specialized activities, which cannot be run by individuals not specifically trained in a subject area, are conducted by paid professionals who occasionally volunteer their services.

There are a number of older adults who eagerly wait at the entrance to our typical center, before the 8:30 opening time, but the majority of the center's members arrive between 10 and 11 A.M. Just inside the entrance, participants, whose sole requirement for participation is having reached age 60, sign in and deposit a coin in a voluntary contribution box. There is no fixed amount, though the average suggested rate for contribution is 30 to 50 cents. The money collected in this manner is used for program enhancement, to add to programs that are not funded directly by the government. How the money is spent is a decision made by elected representatives of the center participants, in conjunction with the center's administrative staff.

Once inside the center, some participants head for formal activities, while others read newspapers or engage in heated discussions, often political, with their colleagues. Still others play cards, hiding the pennies they bet with, for gambling is illegal in the center.

At 12:30 P.M., lunch is served. The hot meal, which is a well-balanced, nutritionally sound one, is served by volunteer participants. Following the meal, all participants are responsible for cleaning up after themselves. Some people begin to head out of the center at this time, while others remain to take part in additional programs. Throughout the day, participants have been meeting with the center director and assistant director for help with their social service needs. The staff, sometimes overburdened by the sheer number of people seeking help, provide information, make referrals, advocate, and counsel to the best of their ability.

The senior citizen center movement, as a result of the variety of services and activities that is offered in centers, has demonstrated that it is of significant value in helping to maintain the social, emotional, and even the physical well-being of older adults. Many centers regularly reevaluate the needs of their participants and attempt to address new needs by instituting new supportive services. Some of the supportive services offered through senior centers will be described in more detail in a later section of this chapter.

Some Difficulties with Senior Citizen Centers. There are many who believe that the senior citizen center movement will continue to grow and expand to meet the changing needs of older persons. There are those, however, who disagree. Senior centers have been referred to as "playpens for the elderly" and accused of providing little more than senior citizen games. These critics point to the fact that centers service less than 20 percent of America's elderly population. Studies indicate that it is not necessarily the fact of participation in senior centers that adds to the quality of life, but rather how active a person is at senior center programs. Those who are the most active tend to have higher levels of self-perceived health, along with greater financial resources (Toseland & Sykes, 1977). It therefore may be those who need services the least who receive most of the assistance offered in senior citizen centers.

These reports are limited, though, and should not be considered typical of all centers. This is not to suggest, however, that senior centers do not have a variety of problems that must be addressed to enhance their effectiveness. Salamon (1981) and Salamon and Trubin (1983) have singled out some general problems and some specific issues which, if reexamined, might add to the overall quality of senior centers. In general, it can be stated that there are four problems that cause difficulties in senior centers:

1. A lack of older-adult investment in the centers
2. Obtrusive rules and regulations governing center programming
3. Inadequate sensitivity to the unique qualities of local communities by regulatory and supervising agencies
4. Overemphasis on providing group meals

All of these problems appear to stem from unnecessary bureaucratic involvement and misunderstanding.

Regarding lack of investment, as we have seen previously, clubs operate successfully based on the principal of balanced reciprocity. Participants give something and hence feel as if they have made an investment. They also get something in return, which serves to increase their subsequent involvement. In some senior citizen centers there exists an "I've got it coming to me" attitude, meaning that an individual just has to show up, does not need to make the voluntary contribution, and can take part in virtually any of the centers' activities. Center directors often complain of the lack of commitment among participants to working on programming issues, and this lack of investment surely is a major contributory factor.

With regard to the problem of obtrusive rules, the federal rules and regulations regarding the operation of senior centers are carried out and interpreted by a number of layers of federal, state, and local government. This intricate network means that the programs in senior centers are subject to much bureaucratic manipulation, further separating older adults from the services they are provided.

Sensitivity to local issues is also a valid issue. Despite a greal deal of difference among the elderly in a variety of communities, there is a tendency by the supervisory organizations to treat all centers the same. There is little effort made to respond to the specific needs of the local community of older adults.

Inadvertently, the government has indeed allocated more funding for the nutritional aspect of senior centers than the other services that are provided. As a result the meals tend to be rather lavish, with only limited social or recreational services available. In locations where there are two or more senior centers within reasonable traveling distance, it is not uncommon for the participants to call all the sites to determine what the luncheon meal will consist of. A decision to attend one of the sites is then made based on the menu and not on any of the other activities or services available.

In addition to these four areas of bureaucratic problems, there is a variety of social interaction problems that trouble senior centers. Meyerhoff (1978), in an in-depth study of one center, found what could be called a sense of emotional urgency: "Ordinary concerns are strangely intense, quickly heating to outburst" (p. 16). She explains the emotional outpourings as resulting from an intense desire to be taken note of before it is too late. Despite this desire to explain it away, it is possible to list at least four types of negative behaviors often seen in senior centers:

1. A refusal to pay, even a minimal amount, for existing and additional services and programs
2. Hoarding of the valued materials of the center, such as eating utensils and arts and crafts supplies
3. Outbreaks of unmannerly behavior
4. Seeking special priveleges at the expense of others

These kinds of behaviors are rarely seen in privately run senior clubs. To overcome these problems and allow for senior centers to expand their service network requires that feelings of reciprocity be generated among participants and between participants and staff. Members should be allowed and encouraged to take active roles in the center, not solely as volunteers with awkward tasks. Their input should be made mandatory and seen as their investment for which they, in return, can anticipate an increasingly strong, responsive center.

SUPPORTIVE SERVICES

A wide variety of services is currently available to help older adults maintain or even improve their quality of life. Often these services exist as part of the programs offered at the local senior citizen center. Sometimes they are sponsored by church and other charity and voluntary associations. Most often these services are supervised by a trained professional, but staffing for the program is made up almost entirely of volunteers, a good many of whom are older adults themselves.

Telephone Reassurance Programs

Often older adults are restricted in their mobility. They find it difficult at times to leave their homes and as a result have limited social contact. A telephone reassurance program is a method of providing regular contact with the restricted older person via the telephone. A trained volunteer or worker will call, sometimes during the day, on a daily basis, for friendly telephone visiting. This contact serves a variety of functions. In addition to being a form of social interaction, the telephone caller acts as a monitor of the health and well-being of the individual called. Should the individual be unable to answer the phone due to illness or accident, the caller will dispatch assistance. If the person called plans to spend a few days away from home, then the worker notes those times. Another function served by the caller is that of information and referral counselor. Should the homebound person require assistance with a human service need, the caller is usually in a position to seek out the proper assistance. Counseling services are sometimes offered via the telephone, and self-help networks may be operated by having some homebound individuals call other persons in a similar situation (Evans & Jaureguy, 1982).

While not considered a direct reassurance program, a system of home emergency monitoring, using the telephone, is a new method of providing for the security of the older person. A variety of systems exists, but all operate on the same general principle: A dailing device is attached to the telephone, and if the older person needs assistance she activates the dialer by pressing or pulling the appropriate button. This system automatically dials a central monitoring station, where a computer identifies the caller and gives the worker vital information, previously recorded, about the caller. On some systems the monitor at the central station can speak directly with the caller. All of this is accomplished without lifting the receiver or dialing the telephone. Once the problem is determined the worker can dispatch the appropriate assistance. While not a substitute for personal contact, these home monitoring systems provide a sense of security not previously available for older adults who live alone.

Widow-to-Widow Groups

Becoming a widow, losing someone you were close with for so many years, can cause extreme emotional stress. Reactions to the loss of a major love object, even when the death is anticipated, are often severe. Some studies indicate a marked deterioration in health within 13 months following the onset of bereavement (Maddision & Viola, 1968). Widowhood results not only in both physical and emotional bereavement reactions, but social and economic as well. Relationships formed with the couple in mind no longer apply (Butler & Lewis, 1976). Friendships based on a partner's associations no longer exist. Financial matters become confusing, particularly when they were in the hands of the dead spouse for so many years.

To help the estimated 13 million widows in the United States, a number of organizations have begun widow-to-widow programs. These self-help programs, often referred to as widowed person's services (Baldwin & Loewinsohn, 1979), offer help to recently widowed individuals. One successful widowed person's service model uses professional counselors and trained peer aides. The aides, themselves widowed, are trained to explore and recognize their own feelings toward widowhood so that they can comfort others experiencing the same emotions. When the widowed person's service is made aware of a new widow, an aide makes an appointment for a visit to the widow. The aide describes the program and suggests how it may be comforting and otherwise helpful. The widow is given a telephone number to call if and when needed and is then allowed to experience his or her own grieving process. Should the widow feel a need for help, the aide may be called. The aide responds by offering emotional support and basic financial advice and often by just sharing a quiet cup of coffee. Should the widow have needs beyond the capabilities of the aide, the aide brings in a professional consultant. Often group counseling and therapy programs evolve as part of widow-to-widow contact.

Some have suggested that the bereavement process is a self-limiting one and that the effects of the loss are generally dealt with constructively in a period of two to three years (Carey, 1979–1980;

Clayton, 1979). Yet the strength of a widow-to-widow service is in making that period of transition an easier one.

Related to the loss of a spouse is the loss of a child, another major area of bereavement that service providers only recently have begun to examine. What little is known about the bereavement process in these situations is limited to the fact that this type of loss is particularly difficult and is rarely overcome (McQuade, 1981). Some widowed person's services have begun to deal with this issue.

Escort and Shopping Services

Transportation is the most important connecting link between home and basic services. Maintaining face-to-face relationships, including shopping, taking part in recreational activities, and visiting the doctor, usually must be done via some means of transportation. In the United States, the private automobile is the primary mode of transportation; however, older adults own fewer automobiles than any other age group, and for them there also is a paucity of any kind of transportation. Public transportation systems do not service many areas, and those that are serviced are usually the major work areas. The public transportation systems that are available usually present a variety of obstacles to their accessibility by older persons. Numerous high steps, unshielded waiting areas, and limited sitting space make it very difficult for an older person to use public means of conveyance (U.S. Senate, 1982). How then, do older adults get around to the services they need?

The government has funded a variety of transportation programs for the elderly. Some of the funds have gone toward renovating public systems to make them more accessible for frailer individuals. Nearly 70 percent of the funds have gone toward dial-a-ride, (Institute of Public Administration, 1975), whereby the older adult calls a central routing office, usually a day or two in advance of need, to request transportation. The dispatcher arranges for the person's ride, usually on a 12-seater minibus, in a taxi, or sometimes on a large school bus.

In certain areas, transportation services are limited to rides to and from health care providers and food shopping. Often transportation is supplemented by an escort service. In addition to transporting the individual, an aide assists the older person in overcoming either physical barriers, such as carrying packages, or language barriers in the maintenance of their service needs. In New York City recently the police department arranged for teenage volunteers to escort older adults on their shopping trips. These escorts go along to assist the older shoppers and also to act as deterrents to potential robbers.

Because many older adults prefer to market for their own grocery needs, the managers of food stores are asked to be mindful of the needs of their elderly customers. Generally, these older shoppers live alone and do not need the large portions of foods packaged for families. A five-pound bag of onions may not only be too heavy for an older person to carry, but it may go to waste. Smaller sizes should be made available for these consumers, and bags should be packed so that each is not too heavy and difficult to carry.

In the provision of these services, it is good to find ways for the recipient to take part in the reciprocity of the system. This may be achieved by allowing tipping of the aides or drivers or by assisting in the planning and routing of the trips. Without this interaction, the program may fail (Matthews, 1982).

Homebound Activity Programs

A friendly visiting service is somewhat analogous to a telephone reassurance program, except that the contact is face-to-face and not over the telephone. In addition to visiting a homebound older adult, the worker may engage in a variety of activities with the homebound person. According to one handbook (Spiller, 1980) an activity may be defined as anything that is engaging, stimulating, challenging, constructive, creative, interesting, and pleasurable. Surely a regular visit relieves the boredom and loneliness experienced by the homebound elderly, but engaging in a task that can be continued following the visit makes it even more worthwhile.

Some homebound activities programs make use of high-school and college volunteers. These volunteers visit the homebound person for about two hours a week. Students who are history majors record the older adults' "living histories." This activity is both a learning experience for the volunteer and a growth experience for the older adult (Halperin, 1981). By speaking of their life experiences, older adults are making the statement that their lives have had an impact. Art students may teach the homebound older adult a new skill. In one instance, a homebound older individual having suffered a stroke on his right and dominant side was shown how to paint with his left hand. His works were so good they were exhibited at a local gallery. Homebound activity programs need not take place exclusively in a home or apartment but may be conducted wherever frail older adults reside without companionship.

Intergenerational Programs

Our culture has minimized the opportunities for the elderly and young to interact. Older adults have a great deal of life experiences to offer youth. Youngsters, on the other hand, need to learn about older adult development. They need to be shown that, apart from the physical changes that take place in the human body over time, the personality of an individual remains relatively stable. To encourage these interactions, a number of older adult service providers have begun a variety of educational and social programs designed to bring together the different generations (Jacobs et al., 1976). Some of those programs have already been mentioned, for example, homebound activities and escort services. Other programs include "rent-a-granny," in which older adults offer their services as babysitters or to assist youngsters with their school work. Other programs include the staging of plays or musical acts by youngsters in senior centers or nursing homes.

To combat the biases of youngsters and the fears they have of old age (Bennett, 1976) a number of educational programs have been established (Ballott, Clark, Fersh, Komanoff, & Patton, 1979; Conte & Salamon, 1981). Three basic approaches have been used:

1. In the *cinematic* approach, students are shown movies and/or slides depicting the lives of the elderly. Discussions inevitably follow.
2. The *didactic* approach uses standard methods of education to impart the salient issues of older adult development, which are often included as part of regular courses.
3. In the *experiential* method, younger students are encouraged to experience things as they would if they were older adults. They are instructed to place cotton in their ears, wear glasses with yellow-tinted or oily lenses, and wear thin rubber gloves on their hands. The students then are asked to attempt to perform a simple home chore, such as threading a needle, counting change, or even opening doors. Students learn firsthand that the external changes do not necessarily change the person within.

ENTITLEMENT PROGRAMS

Entitlements are funds that individuals have a legal right to receive after having fulfilled a certain minimal requirement. Such programs include Social Security and retirement pension funds, low-income assistance, and medical insurance. In this section, we will examine the entitlement programs run by the federal government, including their origins and how effective they presently are in assisting older adults.

Social Security and Supplemental Security Income

In 1935, during the Great Depression, the U.S. Congress passed the Social Security Act. When most people speak about Social Security, they refer to social insurance available to workers at retirement. Social Security however, now encompasses all the major provisions of government insurance, including

- Aid to dependent children and survivors
- Protective service programs
- Public assistance programs

The original designers of the Social Security Act intended to develop a social insurance with compulsory participation for all Americans. The insurance is now designed to provide a minimum amount of protection to all workers and their families in case of inability to work or in the event of death. The program is financed by contributions made both by workers and their employers, all of whom pay amounts to the Social Security fund. The amounts are a proportion of a worker's overall salary. In 1982, 6.7 percent of a worker's earnings up to $32,400 were contributed. Initially, the fund was established as an old-age insurance program covering workers in the industry and commerce fields. In the 1950s and 1960s, agricultural workers, state and local civil servants, and the self-employed were brought into the system.

Social Security provides retirement benefits based on earnings over a worker's lifetime. The more paid in, the higher the payment at retirement. Under the program, payments are made to the worker or the worker's spouse, at retirement age. In the case of survivor's insurance, however, those families with greater need receive somewhat higher benefits. Disability insurance paid between $122.00 and $966.00 per month in 1981; dependent survivors received checks on a monthly basis ranging from $183.00 to $1,120.00; retirement benefits ranged from $98.00 to $500.00. The variability in amounts depends on the number of years worked—and hence contributions made—and the number of dependent family members. Amounts are adjusted regularly to reflect changes in the cost of living.

Most Social Security beneficiaries have more than one source of income; however, Social Security is the major income source for over 60 percent of the elderly in America.

Public Assistance

For those individuals who do not have sufficient financial resources to get by, even with Social Security benefits, public assistance, funded jointly by federal and state governments and administered through local Social Security Administration offices, is available. In 1972, the Social Security Administration was mandated to enact this Supplemental Security Income (SSI) program. The SSI program, which actually started in 1974, was designed to

1. Eradicate the welfare stigma of public assistance.
2. Provide a sense of uniformity in benefits available.
3. Assist the financially destitute, aged, blind, and disabled.

In 1981, if a single person earned $265.00 or less per month and a couple $337.00 per month, they were eligible for SSI. Income is determined by a formula that takes into account the person's living expenses. The federal government encourages states to supplement the SSI benefits to provide higher income for these individuals.

In 1981 almost two million older persons received SSI payments. While this is a large number of people, it is lower than the three to four million initially assumed to need the assistance. One reason for the lowered number of SSI recipients is the possibility that, despite the large outreach effort, a good many elderly individuals are still unaware of the SSI program. Another more likely reason is that many older persons are aware of the program but refuse to apply for benefits. There is still a stigma attached to what is essentially seen as a welfare program (U.S. Senate, 1982).

Housing Assistance

The most recent survey of home ownership performed by the U.S. Bureau of the Census (1980) indicated that nearly 72 percent of those aged 65 and older, who head up households, own their own homes. The ability to keep up these homes, which are primarily in urban areas, and generally over 40 years old, puts a major strain on the older adult. Houses tend to be too large, to be difficult to heat and cool, and to contain a myriad of obsolete equipment in need of repairs. Often these large homes contain a single older person living alone. Nevertheless, residing in one's own home is an important aspect in maintaining one's independence and self-esteem. Society has just begun to realize the value and importance of supporting older adults in their independence by helping them to remain in their own communities and dwellings.

In real terms, older adults tend to have lower housing expenses than other age groups. The proportion of their income spent on housing, however, is higher: As much as 48 percent of an older adult's income may be used for rent or mortgage and maintenance. The Federal Housing Assistance Program, Section 8, was implemented as a means of providing rental assistance for low-income individuals. Close to two million apartments are currently subsidized under this program, and almost 50 percent of them are apartments where the elderly reside. Most states also have rent subsidy programs that help to keep the cost of apartment rental down for older adults, and states or municipalities with colder climates have programs that assist older adults in paying the heating costs of their homes or apartments. In New York State, for example, poor people, regardless of their age group, are entitled to credit for part of the cost of home heating fuel. This Home Energy Assistance Program offers great relief to older adults, particularly those who can show that they spend 30 percent or more of their income on home energy.

Health Insurance

Nearly 70 percent of the entire population have some form of health insurance to cover a portion of the costs for their medical and surgical care (Somers & Somers, 1977). These programs are provided through private insurers such as Blue Cross/Blue Shield and Health Insurance Plan. Many older adults, however, because they are retired and are not eligible for medical insurance coverage normally funded by an employer, and because they cannot afford to pay for this coverage on their own, find themselves without the benefits of health insurance. Before 1965, when Congress enacted Medicare, less than 30 percent of all health care costs were paid for with public funds. The funding at that time consisted primarily of medical public assistance and state and local hospital funds. Following the enactment of government insurance, the government began funding nearly 90 percent of all hospital costs for those over the age of 65. The government program has taken a great burden off older adults in guaranteeing to meet a large measure of their medical costs.

Medicare. The *Medicare* program is funded in the same manner as social security. Workers pay for the insurance which is available to them upon retirement, or in case of disability, through the same annual contributions made to social security. One need not, however, have contributed to social security in order to be eligible for Medicare. The sole requirement for non-disabled individuals is reaching age 65.

Medicare consists of two parts. *Part* A, the hospital insurance portion, pays for inpatient hospital and follow-up care. The medical insurance part, *Part B*, helps pay for physician expenses, certain outpatient hospital procedures and some medical items needed for the maintenance of health. Levels of funding assistance and other provisions of the Medicare program change frequently. The most recent changes (Collins, 1982) include increasing deductibles. Thus, patients now have to pay approximately the first $300.00 of their hospital bills and the first $75.00 for physicians services each year.

Medicaid. Older adults with low incomes are eligible for further health care insurance through a program usually referred to as Medicaid.

Medicaid is funded jointly by both the Federal and State governments. It is, however, administered by the state's public welfare programs. Medicaid, mandated under Title XIX of the Social Security Act, provides for hospital and physician expenses, prescription drugs, nursing home care, and a variety of affiliated health care needs. Almost 50% of all people in nursing homes are covered by Medicaid. Acceptance for reimbursement under Medicaid requires an inspection of financial resources referred to as a "*means test.*" The means test is performed to verify that all other financial resources available to older adults have been expended. Despite the fact that many older adults have moderate illnesses which can exhaust their finances, a good many older persons refuse to succumb to a means test. Not only is the acceptance of welfare support seen as insulting, but the means test is sometimes seen as degrading.

There have been some recent funding changes in Medicaid which like Medicare also affect the program's ability to assist older people. Federal cutbacks of funds to the states may cause a state to re-evaluate how best to allocate its own financial resources. Particularly in states where there may be economic difficulties, it is anticipated that there will be major cutbacks in allocations for medical cost assistance.

Private Insurance for Older Adults. Recently a number of insurance companies have begun to make available a variety of health insurance programs tailored specifically for older persons. Because of the wide variety and questionable nature of some of them, it is important to examine each program carefully and determine if the increased coverage is necessary.

Food Stamps

Another entitlement program available to financially strapped older adults is food stamps. The program, enacted in 1964, allows individuals to purchase food with government coupons. Food is a major expense that takes an ever increasing bite from the older adults' resources. Many peoples' income leaves them precious little with which to buy food, after rent, utilities, and other necessities have been paid for. It is no wonder that there have been horror stories of older adults eating dog food! Food stamps allow low-income individuals to purchase the necessary staples for life. Of the 22.5 million Americans receiving food stamps in 1981, only 10 percent were older adults. Eligibility for food stamps is established at the federal level and is regularly reevaluated. It is dependent upon the amount of income and number of individuals who share a household. One distressing problem recently noted is that, due to recent changes in the SSI funding regulations, individuals receiving food stamp assistance may be declared to be earning too much to be eligible to continue to receive SSI benefits.

Fiscal Problems

Government entitlement programs serve the needs of a good many older persons, but programs so large and with so much beauracratic involvement tend to have a variety of problems. A seemingly insurmountable problem recently brought to the attention of the public is the dwindling of the government's Social Security fund. One reason for the lower fund reserve is the poor growth performance of the economy. The fund is actually three separate trust funds: old age and survivor's insurance, disability insurance, and hospital insurance. The only fund with a current serious economic problem is the old age and survivor's insurance. To overcome this problem, interfund borrowing was instituted. It is expected, however, that, with the projected increase in hospital costs and the ever growing number of elderly people, the three funds may not have sufficient resources. A number of suggestions have been made to help overcome this problem. Among them are lowering the amount of benefits made available, taking funds from the general economy, and tying the funding to a new tax method.

Other fiscal problems are related to government-sponsored health insurance and related benefits, and these are even more disturbing. There have been cases of widespread fraud and abuse noted, particularly in the Medicaid system (U.S. Senate, 1982). In many cases, untrustworthy health care providers have billed for services not provided.

Some interesting gaps in medical insurance coverage exist. One glaring example is that Medicare will pay for an older adult's visit to an ophthalmologist for an eye examination; however, should the physician prescribe a new set of glasses, generally more expensive than the cost of the visit to the doctor, the individual must find a way to purchase the glasses without assistance. Medicare does not reimburse for that expense, nor does it reimburse for hearing aids, dental care, or hospice services.

A major complaint regarding Medicaid is that it is heavily weighted toward institutional care. If medical and health care services are provided to older adults in their own homes by family members, there is no reimbursement under Medicaid. If the services are provided in the home by a licensed health professional, only some states will allow for reimbursement. If the services are performed in a nursing home, the fees are covered in their entirety (U.S. Senate, 1982).

SUMMARY

This chapter has described the importance of social service programs in the lives of older adults, and we have taken a look at the support systems of older adults, both formal and informal. We also examined the various forms of government-funded pensions, benefits, and health insurance programs available to older persons. We now turn to a detailed look at health care, a subject of major importance in the lives of most older adults.

2

Health Care Programs and Options for Care

At any given time, only about 5 percent of all people over the age of 65 live in nursing homes, yet most older people have at least one chronic illness. The elderly, because of their high rates of illness, are major clients of a variety of health care programs, not simply institutionally based ones. In 1983, older adults represented roughly 12 percent of the population of the United States, while close to 30 percent of national health care expenditures, representing personal health care costs, went toward the health care of older Americans. While $13 billion was spent on nursing home care, $49 billion was spent for other health care expenses provided to elderly people living in the community (U.S. Senate, 1985). In this chapter, we will look at the variety of health care services available to older adults, both for the community resident and the individual requiring institutionalization. We will not deal with specific physical ailments or emotional problems. We will, however, look at institutionalized health care services and the needs to which they were designed to respond.

LEVELS OF PREVENTION

Health care intervention traditionally has been divided into three levels: primary, secondary, and tertiary prevention. At the first level, that of *primary prevention*, the goal of the health care provider is to prevent illness by reducing an individual's exposure to an "at-risk" situation. Programs offered in senior centers whereby older adults learn how to prevent accidents from occurring in their homes or apartments would be included in this category.

Secondary prevention is directed toward minimizing the progression of illness and disease by screening, early detection, and prompt direct treatment. Hospital-sponsored health screening fairs where tests are given for glaucoma, diabetes, and high blood pressure, among others, are considered one aspect of secondary prevention. If an illness is discovered, the person is referred for treatment.

The third level of intervention occurs when an illness has become serious. *Tertiary prevention* seeks to limit the disability and restore functioning as much as possible.

TYPES OF CARE

As noted previously, health care services can be provided in a variety of settings. Here too, however, it is useful to distinguish three types of care: inpatient, outpatient, community care. Inpatient services are provided in an institution for residents of the institution. Outpatient services also are provided in health facilities, but in this case it is for community residents who travel to the institution to receive their care. Community care is provided in the community for those residents who are essentially healthy. Examples include annual checkups, dental visits, and eye examinations.

THE INTERFACE: CHOICES FOR HEALTH CARE

The three types of health care and the three levels of prevention are presented visually in Figure 2–1. The level of prevention is represented on the vertical axis, while the type of service is provided is displayed on the horizontal axis. The third axis shows the levels of care available. At the level where an individual is quite ill and requires total rehabilitation care in an inpatient facility, the choice for care will probably be a hospital or nursing home. As you move toward decreasing levels of need, more options become available. Home care, for example, may be substituted for individuals who normally require round-the-clock monitoring but not necessarily round-the-clock skilled nursing supervision. Adult day care may be used by an individual who requires daily health care monitoring but not on a 24-hour basis.

The way choices for health care are made by older adults when options are available depends on a number of important issues related to the needs of the patient, the involvement of the patient's family, government entitlements, and the health care provider. One major

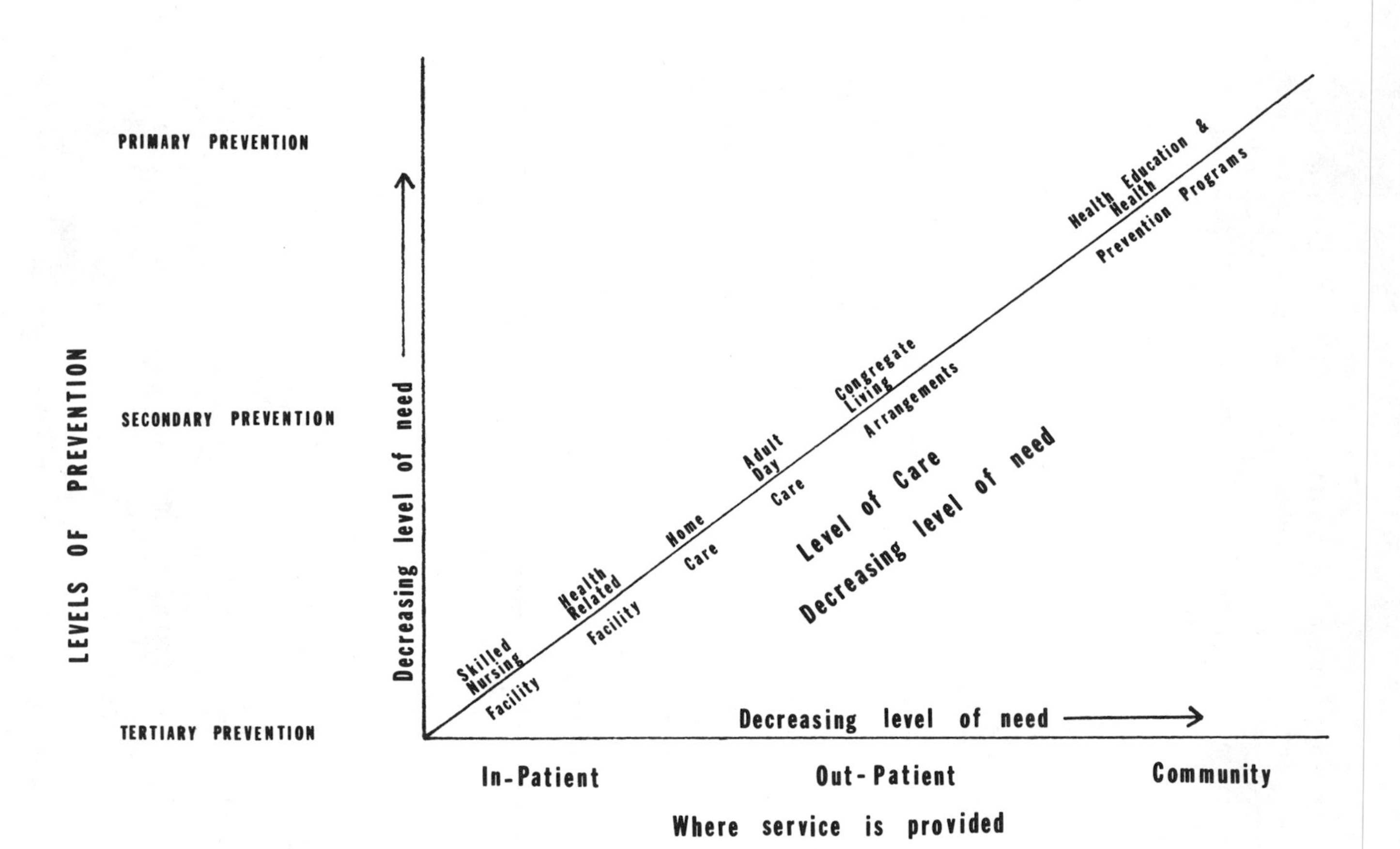

Figure 2–1 The Three Axes of Care.

issue for the older patient in choosing what type of care they wish to receive generally relates to quality of life. Many older adults find it difficult to survive in the community while attending to their failing physical needs. They may realize that remaining in the community promises them increasing loneliness, isolation, and separation from services, and so they may elect to enter a retirement home or some other residential facility.

The amount of social support available from family and neighbors is also a critical factor in making the decision to move to an institution. The family may want to maintain an older adult in her own apartment but may find it difficult to do so. The family may be monetarily strapped, or both spouses have to work, making it difficult to find the time to visit and care for the older adult. They may even have offered the older parent the opportunity to move in with them. That alternative may not be considered a viable one, however, for there is no one at home during the day and there are few older adults in the community where the family resides. Another consideration, is that the older person's already meager SSI benefits will be cut by one-third if she moves to her children's home.

Whenever a difficult choice such as this must be made, the decision should be based on both the instrumental or objective health care needs and the affective or emotional–social needs of the individual requiring the care. Often, however, health care providers tend to evaluate their older-adult patients solely in a mechanistic, instrumental fashion. Often this is the result of a negative attitude on the part of the physician toward the elderly (Salamon, 1979; Strain, 1981), whereby the aging process quickly becomes equated with deterioration and death. Even among physicians, the popular misconception that illness is a normal part of aging is perpetuated. Most doctors prefer to deal with younger individuals who have less chronic diseases and are therefore more likely to be cured. The medical problems presented by the elderly tend to be more difficult, and the demands older adults place on the care provider are more intense. The reaction of the doctor is sometimes to treat the older person in an infantile manner and recommend a level of care not totally warranted. While this does not occur constantly, it occurs with sufficient frequency to warrant wariness. It is important to guard against the deleterious effects that may result from these biased behaviors.

In most cases, a person's decision as to the type of care he should receive and where the care will be obtained is made after careful consideration of all the known options. In this chapter we will discuss some of the better-known options and take a closer look at some of the new programs that have been developed.

HEALTH-EDUCATION AND RECREATION PROGRAMS

A couple of anecdotes will help to illustrate an important issue in health education. One concerns an older woman who came into the senior center nurse's office with a lunch-size brown paper bag that was obviously quite full. The nurse was at the center to monitor blood pressures, volunteering her time one morning a month. The woman sat down, and the nurse took her blood pressure. The nurse told the woman it was a little high. The woman said "I thought so, I haven't been feeling too well lately," and proceeded to empty the contents of the paper bag onto the nurse's desk. The woman went on to explain that her husband had died five years previously and that these medications were his. She had saved them in the refrigerator. Now that she was not feeling well, she wondered if she might be able to take any of these medicines. The nurse explained that even if the medications were the correct ones they had already expired so they would have to be disposed of.

On another occasion, two men were having lunch at a senior center. Following the meal, one of the men complained of severe intestinal pain. His friend offered him a pill for angina pain, which he took.

While these anecdotes may sound farfetched, they are real and, unfortunately, did take place. They point to just one of the major misconceptions older adults have regarding their health needs, namely, the proper use of medications. The poor eating and exercise habits of the elderly also contribute to lower levels of health. To cope with these illness-oriented behaviors, a variety of recreational and educational programs have been developed. An overview of these programs will be presented here, while the categories of programs and specific activities will be discussed in greater detail in chapter 7.

Behavior and Attitude

Maintaining good health and receiving the appropriate health care services are essential to an older adult's good quality of life. Yet many older adults exhibit a wide variety of inappropriate or poor behavior, including

- Poor nutrition
- Lack of exercise
- Lack of compliance with prescribed medication regimens
- Postponement of seeking appropriate medical services
- Misuse of those services that are obtained

There is also a poor understanding of the aging process among many older adults themselves. Older persons often fail to understand that many of their physical complaints may in fact be due to disease processes that are not part of normal aging. There is widespread misunderstanding as to the proper use of medications, both over the counter and prescribed. An additional problem older adults often have is a negative attitude, exemplified by the feeling that illness is part of one's fate and therefore inevitable. If that is thought to be valid, then what follows is that the disease becomes untreatable.

An even more common attitude among the elderly is an inability or unwillingness to question the health care provider. For example, a physician may prescribe a drug for high blood pressure, and the older adult may not ask about side-effects, nor may the physician offer the information. If the side-effects do occur, the older person may stop the medication without consulting the doctor.

Program Goals

Health-education programs seek to teach older adults about the issues most important to them. By teaching about the aging process and specific disease states, and by helping to change attitudes and clarify beliefs, health-education programs seek to reach their goal of health maintenance. The goal is twofold. First, not only is an individual helped to remain healthy, but the drain on health care resources and medical services is minimized. Another important goal is to eliminate the estimated $2 billion spent annually by the elderly on medical products that are useless. Quack medicines advertised as miracle cures for arthritis and cancer promise older adults relief that their physicians cannot provide. The promise of a cure, lower fees, and friendly sales representatives all contribute to the continuation of these snake-oil practices (Ducovney, 1969). Health educators carefully explain disease processes and treatment methods, in order to make older adults more aware of fraudulant schemes.

The Educational Process

The programs that provide health education for older adults tend to be community oriented and disease specific. These programs, such as exercises for arthritis, often are sponsored by hospital or local health groups. The programs are offered to individuals who have been identified as being at risk. The programs generally use screening, lectures, and distribution of pamphlets and other reading materials in their educational approach. The progression of the disease, along with its symptoms, are discussed; treatment modalities are examined; and sometimes the feelings of those who have the illness are explored. The educational material used generally comes from governmental sources and nonprofit organizations such as the National Heart Association, American Cancer Society, Blue Cross/Blue Shield, and other similar groups.

A number of organizations have begun to prepare comprehensive educational programs designed for older adults. Among these are Healthwise of Idaho and the program sponsored by the Mountain States Health Corporation (Gaarder & Cohen, 1982). These organizations have found that, despite the fact that many health professionals have difficulty dealing with the elderly, older adults eagerly participate in health-education programs (German, 1978). Not only is there specific interest on older persons' parts regarding issues directly related them, but the elderly often express a desire to assume more responsibility for their own health care needs.

In order for a health-education program to be successful, it should follow a number of basic steps:

1. Education should be offered by a variety of methods, not just through lectures.
2. There should be frequent discussions, and exercises should be used when appropriate.
3. It is important to have the activity in a room that is well ventilated and poses limited distractions, particularly noise.
4. The participants themselves should be asked to contribute to the educational process. This should be done both by asking them to state their objectives and what they would like to accomplish and by preparing a brief presentation, if appropriate.
5. Self-care goals also should be established. These include breast self-examination, blood pressure monitoring, and other self-activated tasks to complement professional care.
6. When a program runs for more than one session, there should be frequent reviews of the material already covered.
7. Most important to the educational needs of the elderly is to treat the participants with the appropriate degree of respect. This includes not talking down to the participants and encouraging a good deal of input.

The use of health professionals is recommended; however, most groups can be run by well-read nonprofessionals. It is also a good idea to have large charts and drawings and a well-situated blackboard.

What follows is an outline of an 11-session health-education program done in a number of senior centers in the New York City area. The sessions were designed to last for two hours, including a 15- to 20-minute break. The progression of topics discussed did not follow any particular order, nor are they comprehensive. This is just one of many possible methods of providing knowledge to older people, to help them maintain a higher level of health. It can provide a useful example of some of the topics worthy of discussion.

Meeting 1: Introduction. At the first meeting, participants are asked to list the issues they wish to discuss and what they hope to gain from the program. An introduction to health education in general and how it may benefit older adults is made. An introduction to the normal aging process, including physical and emotional changes, is presented.

Meeting 2: Circulation. An overview of the human circulatory system is provided. Common circulatory diseases are discussed, along with the disease process and methods of treatment. How to recognize some of these disorders is an important part of the discussion. There is also an introduction to the function of the heart.

Meeting 3: The Auditory System. The intricate structure and functions of the auditory system are explained. Some illnesses of the ear are reviewed. The importance of properly cleaning away ear wax is stressed. The use of hearing aids and the emotional impact they may have are explored.

Meeting 4: Choosing and Communicating with a Doctor. This is a topic in which all participants had a great deal of interest. The importance of finding a physician who one feels comfortable with is stressed, as are ways of looking for specialists and doctors who know how to listen well. Ways to evaluate the way a doctor performs an examination are discussed, as well as general questions to ask your doctor, particularly when a form of treatment is prescribed.

Meeting 5: Medications. The difference between brand-name and generic drugs is discussed, and a list of essential home medicines is reviewed. The major drug interactions to be avoided are presented. How to use over-the-counter drugs, the importance of maintaining a prescribed drug regimen, and when to speak to a doctor or pharmacist regarding the side-effects of medications are all part of this session.

Meeting 6: Coronary Illness. Shortness of breath resulting from coronary insufficiencies is discussed, and heart failures are explored in detail. Drugs that strengthen the heart, special diets, and the importance of exercise are all examined.

Meeting 7: Pulmonary Disease. Shortness of breath due to pulmonary changes is discussed. The combined importance of lungs and heart for oxygen transfer is explained. Treatments of common ailments such as chronic obstructive heart disease, bronchitis, asthma, and other disorders of the lung are reviewed. The meaning of spots on the lung is also reviewed.

Meeting 8: Stomach. The effects of aging on the digestive process are explained. How dentures can affect the digestive process and the affects of different food preferences are all explored. Common digestive difficulties, including heartburn, hiatus hernia, and ulcers, are discussed.

Meeting 9: Bowels. The importance of balanced nutrition is explained. There is a detailed discussion of regularity and normal bowel movements. How to treat hemorrhoids and detect cancer of the bowel is reviewed.

Meeting 10: Weakness and Dizziness. The importance of seeing these factors as emanating from illnesses and not normal aging is stressed. Anemia and other blood problems are explained, along with thyroid disease, middle-ear problems, heart disease, and tumors, as possible causes of the symptoms.

Meeting 11: Emotional Well-being. A discussion of the stressfulness of certain life events is conducted. Ways of reducing stress and preparing for specific unavoidable events are explored. Participants are taught to recognize when professional help is indicated. Overcoming the stigma of getting professional psychotherapeutic help and where to get that assistance are reviewed.

For health-education programs to become effective, emphasis must be placed on the benefits of health promotion and illness prevention. Currently, while there has been some movement in this direction (New York State, 1980) most health care cost-reimbursement programs fund exclusively for health care, not illness prevention. One of the benefits of health-education programs is to lower overall health care expenditures by teaching older adults to take better care of themselves. It is important for us to view the positive aspects of these programs in future policy planning.

HEALTH CARE FOR COMMUNITY RESIDENTS

The majority of older persons prefer to maintain an independent existence within their community and in an apartment of their own (Carp, 1977; Shanas, 1971). Most are capable of doing so with only a limited amount of help (Butler & Lewis, 1976; Moon, 1983), most of which comes from social support networks—both informal, from family and friends, and formal, from social service providers. The types of services needed by the home dwelling elderly vary according to their physical state. Needs may range from a once-yearly physical in a physician's office to round-the-clock nursing supervision. This section will review the most common health care options available to older adults, according to their medical need. We will examine a variety of options ranging from private practitioner visits to occasional use of an acute-care hospital. Other, more unusual options, such as adult day-care and geriatric foster care, where older adults are maintained in the community, will be examined in a later section entitled "Innovative Programs."

Physicians' Offices

Most people have their own family physician. This physician is a person they have known and felt confident with for many years. As people age, however, the use of this one, trusted doctor dwindles, for a variety of reasons. As people age so do their physicians. Some of these doctors retire. There is information that indicates that those who do remain in practice may not be as likely as their younger colleagues to remain as actively abreast of new developments in the field (Kovar, 1980). Often older adults relocate to new neighborhoods. Family members sometimes recommend the use of a different physician to the older adult. Also, the use of numerous specialists increases with age. Despite the changes that take place, older adults visit office-based doctors more often than any other age group. The average number of visits to a doctor for the general population is under five visits per year. For an older adult the average number of visits per year is greater than six. One obvious reason is that older people are twice as likely as younger individuals to have a chronic condition. As a result they visit internists more frequently than other age groups and have more tests, such as blood pressure readings and electrocardiograms, performed than younger individuals. There are no reliable figures as to how often older adults call physicians or whether their doctors make house calls. Most physicians do not make house calls, although there are indications that this may be changing (U.S. Senate, 1982).

Some difficulties exist in the use of office-based physicians for older adults. Particularly for older individuals who rely on medical insurance, the cost of a visit to a private practitioner may be prohibitive. Office-based physicians may well accept the medical insurance of an older adult as only partial payment of their higher fee. Under Medicare, if a physician accepts "assignment," Medicare will pay 80 percent of the allowable expenses directly to the physician. The patient is responsible for the remaining 20 percent.

Another issue related to office-based care is the lack of physicians trained in geriatric medicine. In fact, the specialty of geriatric medicine is still not widely accepted in America. Misconceptions regarding the normal health needs of the older adult are still widespread among doctors. In a recent survey of the medical schools in America, less than 10 percent indicated an interest in formally teaching geriatric medicine to their medical students (Moss & Halamandaris, 1977).

Older adults who do not have a physician they consider their own tend to use the service of the local hospital emergency room or clinic. In most hospital-affiliated and private clinics, the medical care older individuals receive is quite adequate, despite the fact that they may not see the same physician more than once. There are, however, scandalous instances of fraud that take place in some clinics, referred to as "Medicaid mills." These clinics will see individuals and accept whatever medical insurance they may have as payment in full. Despite the fact that the reimbursement rates of programs such as Medicare and Medicaid are low, the clinic will not ask for additional fees. The older patient sees this as a blessing. To compensate for the lower income per patient, physicians in the Medicaid mill spend less time with each patient in order to see more patients, and they order more medical tests to be performed than normally would be warranted (Thompson, 1980). Furthermore, the patient might be referred to another physician within the clinic, even if it is not necessary, to bring in still more consultation fees. Though there have been cases of patient mistreatment in these establishments, in general the medical care is at least average. What has to be managed is the amount of waste, in terms of effort, money, and time, that occurs in these places. To do that requires a reevaluation of the medical insurance reimbursement scheme (Thompson, 1980).

Dental Care

About half of all Americans visit a dentist once a year. Less than 30 percent over the age of 65, however, do so. Of those who do go, older adults go for an average of only slightly more than one time per year, while all other age groups go at least twice. One reason that has been advanced for the lowered rates is to loss of teeth. It is estimated that over 45 percent of those over the age of 65 have lost most or all of their own teeth. Many older persons who have few of their own teeth believe that they do not need to see a dentist. On the contrary, toothlessness can affect their ability to eat a wide variety of nutritionally sound foods and thus can cause nutrition-related illnesses. Dentist visits are therefore recommended, even for those older adults who have full dentures.

Another reason why older adults do not visit dentists regularly is their financial status. Most medical insurance programs do not cover the cost of regular dental care. It has been reported that, of those older persons who do see dentists, 97 percent of the cost for their oral care comes out of their own pockets. This is in sharp contrast to the 29 percent of costs paid out of pocket for regular medical care by the elderly.

Short-stay Hospitals

Both elderly residents of the community and those elderly who reside in institutions make use of short-stay, acute-care hospitals. When they show signs of developing acute illnesses, or when the chronic illnesses they already have enter an acute phase, a hospital is generally the appropriate facility for treatment. Older persons have almost twice as many hospital stays as younger persons. Once they are in the short-term acute-care hospital, older adults average close to 12 days per visit, twice as long as younger people. One measure of hospital usage is discharge rate. Those individuals between the ages of 64 and 84 have a discharge rate twice as high as all other age groups. Individuals over the age of 85 have a hospital discharge rate that is even higher, 70 percent above the 64-to-84 age group (Federal Council on the Aging, 1981).

Current Trends. An examination of the use of hospitals by the elderly over the past 30 years has shown a number of trends:

1. Older men tend to be hospitalized more frequently than women.
2. As a result of the introduction of Medicare, the poorer and minority elderly tend to use short-stay hospitals almost as frequently as nonminority elderly. This is in contrast to the lower rate of utilization of hospitals by the poor and minority elderly prior to the inception of Medicare.
3. Elderly people also are more likely to be hospitalized than they were before the introduction of Medicare. There is, though, a slight reduction in the average number of days spent in the hospital (Brehm, 1980).

Hospital Biases. Once older adults enter an acute-care hospital, they are sometimes misdirected or inappropriately cared for. Butler

(1975) has described some of the strategies hospital personnel use to deal with older patients. One technique, which is employed in the emergency room, is referred to as the *emergency room hustle*. The patient receives only a cursory examination, is told that everything appears normal for a person of that age, and is sent home.

Some voluntary hospitals play what is known as the *transfer game*. Because the hospital prefers patients who are able to pay privately, older-adult Medicare patients are transferred to a public hospital. When transfers like this go on indefinitely, the strategy is called the *shuttle*. The public hospital may be overburdened and have no room for additional patients, so a second transfer is performed. There have been reports of transfers like this going on to the point where patients have died in the ambulance. Luckily, attention has been drawn to these issues and changes have been instituted.

Most older patients do receive proper treatment in acute-care hospitals. Once discharged, however, the majority of these individuals return to the community, to their own homes and apartments, and most still need medical attention and assistance with skills of daily living.

Home Health Assistants

Depending on the need of the individual older adult, a variety of options for health care in the home exists. There are several reasons why older individuals choose to receive their care at home:

1. Obviously, there is fear of institutionalization. The common feeling among older adults is, "Once you enter a nursing home the only way you come out is in a pine box." As we shall see shortly, the figures bear this out.
2. There is a desire to remain in familiar surroundings, an added feature of which is the sense of independence one feels when at home.
3. Home health care services may be less expensive than institutional care (U.S. General Accounting Office, 1978; New York Business Group, 1982).

The services provided at home for older adults can be grouped into two categories, support with activities of daily living and professional services. The supportive personal services usually are provided by specially trained homemakers. Professional services are provided by nurses, rehabilitation specialists, and supervised paraprofessionals.

Homemakers. Generally, these people are professionally supervised to provide supportive services to homebound older adults. They undergo a basic training program to acquaint them with the needs of their clients and how to cope with some common problems of illness in the homebound elderly. A homemaker, however, is not a substitute for a nurse. A homemaker's duties are to shop, clean, prepare meals, do light chores, and be a friendly companion.

Home Health Aides. Paraprofessional nursing care is provided in older adults' homes by home health aides. Their services are covered by Medicare, whereas homemakers' fees are not. Therefore, in a number of communities the role of the homemaker and home health aide are combined. The role of the home health aide is to assist with the personal hygiene needs of the client, give medications, and assist with physical therapy.

Professional Care. Professional nursing is also provided in some communities for the ill or recuperating homebound elderly. Under programs such as the Visiting Nurse Service, trained nurses, who also act as case supervisors, coordinate all the home health care needs of their elderly patients. These services include changing dressings and giving other treatments; supervising the home health aide and the physical, occupational, and speech therapists; requesting social services; and ordering surgical supplies and equipment.

While there is strong debate on this issue, it is estimated that as many as one-quarter of the elderly who are presently institutionalized would be better cared for in their own homes (Carp, 1977). It also has been estimated that 2.5 million elderly individuals are in need of home health care but, due to a shortage of workers, are doing without these services (Moss & Halmandaris, 1977). It also has been correctly suggested that older adults who are terminally ill could live their remaining days in greater dignity if they had the proper support at home, rather than in cold, institutional settings. Little wonder that the Technical Committee on Family, Social Services and Other Support Systems of the White House Conference on Aging (1981) has urged expanding the services that enable older adults to remain in their own homes when that is the best alternative.

HEALTH-RELATED OR INTERMEDIATE-CARE FACILITIES

In instances where 24-hour supervision is necessary and cannot be provided in the older adults' own home or apartment, a move to an institutional residence may be indicated. There are generally two types of institutional facilities that provide ongoing health care for the elderly: (1) a skilled nursing facility or nursing home, which we will discuss in the next section, and (2) a health-related facility or intermediate-care facility.

As the name implies, a health-related or intermediate-care facility provides round-the-clock care, but at an intermediate level of medical supervision. In most instances, one registered or professional nurse is required to supervise the health care of all the residents. The actual care is performed by licensed professional nurses and nurse's aides.

The level of illness of the residents of the health-related facility is moderate. Most individuals in the facility are not very ill, though all have a chronic health problem requiring monitoring. The residents are generally ambulatory, though they may need therapy to restore and rehabilitate themselves to a previous level of functioning. The therapy to accomplish this is offered in an intermediate-care facility. Other services generally provided in a health-related facility include recreation, counseling, education, arts and crafts, and hair grooming.

The intermediate-care facility should not be confused with what used to be referred to as an "old-age home." The old-age home generally was a hotel to which older adults would retire, renting their own rooms and coming and going as they pleased. This is not the case in a health-related or intermediate-care facility, where there are medical requirements for admission and restrictions regarding leaving the facility. The old-age home, now replaced by the domiciliary care facility or adult home, is generally licensed and supervised by a state department of public welfare, whereas health-related facilities are licensed by state departments of health. The costs of residing in a domiciliary care facility are borne by Social Security and Supplemental Security Income, whereas the health-related facility costs are reimbursed under Medicare. Typically, its residents are individuals who may be suffering mild confusion, are recovering from a moderate stroke or heart attack, or are simply too frail to live alone in their own homes. Individuals whose level of functioning indicates that they need a higher level of health care and supervision are placed in a nursing home when no other alternative exists.

SKILLED NURSING FACILITIES

Demographics

A nursing home or skilled nursing facility (SNF) cares for individuals who are quite ill. The average patient in a nursing home has a variety of health problems, takes an average of four different medications daily, is often—almost 70 percent of the time—semi- or nonambulatory, is older and more socially isolated than the average nonresident, and is frequently disoriented and confused. It has been estimated that roughly 50 percent of nursing home residents are senile, though that is probably an inaccurate diagnosis (Vladeck, 1980). The individual patient in a nursing home requires intensive, ongoing medical supervision.

SNF's are one of the most costly forms of ongoing medical care available, and the costs are rising at a rate that is almost 2 percent higher than other health services. This annual rate, almost 17 percent, may end up jeopardizing other services for older adults because of the large chunk it takes from the Medicare/Medicaid pie (U.S. Senate, 1982).

The population of elderly SNF residents has increased rapidly in the past two decades. In 1963, there were slightly more than half a million patients residing in nursing homes. In 1980, that amount jumped to almost 1.5 million (Brehm, 1980). One reason for this sharp rise is the institution of Medicare, which guarantees payments for nursing home care. Based on population estimates and types of care needed, it has been suggested that, by the year 2000, another half a million nursing home beds will be needed to accommodate the increasing number of elderly (Brehm, 1980).

Eighty six percent of the residents of nursing homes are over the age of 65. While this is approximately 5 percent of the population over 65, the likelihood of requiring nursing home care increases with age, as does the need for all other health services. Between the ages of 65 and 74, the rate of institutionalization in an SNF is 1.2 percent. The figure rises to almost 7 percent between ages 75 and 84, and more than triples to almost 22 percent for individuals over age 85 (Vladeck, 1980).

The average age of SNF patients is 82, and typically they are widowed women. Almost 22 percent of nursing home residents were never married, 5 percent are divorced, and only about 10 percent have a living spouse. Almost half of nursing home residents have no living relatives, and more than 60 percent do not have regular visitors. The prognosis for discharge from the SNF to one's own home or an intermediate-care facility is much better for those who do have a spouse. Only 20 percent, however, will return home. The vast majority of nursing home residents die in the facility or in a hospital they have been transferred to from the skilled nursing facility (Moss & Halamandaris, 1977; Federal Council on the Aging, 1981).

In a number of cases, it is important to provide care for older adults outside of their own homes or apartments. These situations include instances where

1. The relative or other informal support giver is limited in the amount of strength, both physical and psychological, available to undertake such a task.
2. The care provider has limited financial resources and must spend a good amount of time outside the home, at work.
3. Poor patient–family relationships exist.
4. There are very young children, or other individuals of the family who need a good deal of attention.
5. The facilities at home are inadequate.
6. The care needs of the older person are extreme.

Perhaps the most difficult decision a family has to make regarding its ill older adult member is deciding on long-term institutionalization.

There are those who have argued that older adults should never require the services of an intermediate-care facility or a skilled nursing facility. The care these individuals require, they believe, could be provided for by family and other supports in the patient's home. They even point to the fact that, before the 1940s nursing homes did not exist. This, however, is a misconception, for the following reasons:

1. Medical science has increased the overall lifespan and made it possible for larger proportions of individuals to live longer lives. Proportionally, there are more older adults alive today than at any previous time in our history.

2. While the advances that caused this longevity were taking place, society has become more urbanized and industrialized. Families are no longer available to assist in the health care of an aged family member around the clock.

3. Our health reimbursement systems encourage institutionalization by not paying for many home health care services. Families not financially well off may find their resources pushed beyond their limits by caring for a family member at home.

4. Further, as we will see, nursing homes serve the needs of a very small, very select group of older, infirm adults.

Nursing homes are not, as commonly portrayed, dumping grounds for old people. Most importantly, there is increasing evidence that some older adults are better off emotionally when cared for in a nursing home than at home (Robinson, 1983; Salamon, 1983a). This may result from the social stimulation that takes place there.

Care in Nursing Homes

Nursing home or SNF care as we know it is a relatively new development. The concept of caring for the elderly in boarding or convalescent homes can be traced back to Colonial times (Vladeck, 1980). However, facilities licensed by health departments and offering nursing rehabilitation services began to appear mostly in the 1930s and 1940s.

Skilled nursing facilities are licensed in all states by the state's department of health and are governed by federal regulations issued from the U.S. Department of Health and Human Services. The federal government pays state licensing agencies to inspect, on a yearly basis, nursing homes that participate in the Medicare and Medicaid programs. Among items inspected are (1) the staff-to-patient ratios, (2) whether or not appropriate rehabilitation therapies are available, and (3) the sanitary conditions.

Doctors in Nursing Homes. There has been a great deal of talk about the type of medical care physicians provide to SNF residents. Doctors are required by Medicare and Medicaid to visit a nursing home resident at least once a month to review the patient's condition and reevaluate the type of care needed. It has been found that physician visits cluster at monthly intervals. This suggests that the visits are seen more as a discharge of responsibility on the part of the physician, rather than as a tool for guaranteeing regular, ongoing medical supervision (Willemain & Mark, 1980).

Not only do physicians visit nursing homes infrequently, but only a small proportion of physicians visit nursing homes at all (Mitchell, 1982). A variety of reasons have been given for this finding. Some doctors may not wish to deal with deteriorated nursing home patients who have only a slim possibility for cure (Kane, Jorgenson, Tireberg, & Kawahora, 1976). The red tape required to receive Medicaid reimbursement is also a strong disincentive (Special Committee on Aging, 1975). The most likely reason, however, is the relatively low reimbursement rates paid by Medicare and Medicaid for nursing home visits. While the rates paid are comparable to office visits, there is no reimbursement for doctors' traveling time and expenses.

Myths and Biases. Increasing the rate of reimbursement may bring more physicians into SNF's but may not change the negative stereotype of the hopeless patient. One means of overcoming that is through education. The federal government recently has funded a variety of educational programs for physicians and nurses using the nursing home as a site for training (U.S. Senate, 1982). This program should go a long way toward upgrading attitudes and physician–patient interactions in the years ahead.

Nursing homes, despite the corruption and poor patient care reported in the recent past, are not generally facilities of abuse. While there are always exceptions to every rule, most facilities attempt to give and succeed in providing a reasonable level of patient care. Patient's rights are carefully observed to make sure that there is no abuse. Most states have oversight organizations that examine even the slightest cases of inappropriate patient care. Also, most nursing homes have resident councils, which are organizations of nursing home residents that make recommendations regarding the care they wish to receive, which are given to the administration of the nursing homes they themselves live in. These councils are designed to give residents the ability to share constructively in decision making and allow them to make a useful contribution to their own community (Silverstone, 1974).

Satisfaction with Care. It is very difficult to determine how satisfied residents of SNF's are with their living arrangements. Some residents may be too confused to respond appropriately. Others may be angry with everything. Still others may be fearful to speak ill of the nursing home for fear of retaliation by facility personnel.

A study performed a few years ago (Kahana, 1975) attempted to ascertain the satisfaction with life among nursing home residents. Kahana surveyed 50 residents from 14 nursing homes in two counties in the state of Michigan. Thirty percent of those surveyed said that life in the nursing home was either moderately good or very positive. A similar proportion, 27 percent, were neutral regarding their level of satisfaction, while 34 percent were negative. Fifty six percent of the residents in the homes surveyed said that the facility was worse than expected. The reasons included a reduced lack of mental stimulation, lack of freedom, and poor food. A large majority of the residents surveyed—92 percent—had no complaints about staff or the care they received from them; however, as stated before, fear of retaliation may account for this high percentage, so it should be viewed with a bit of skepticism.

In a more recent study (Salamon, 1983a), 241 patients in a variety of nursing homes and intermediate-care facilities, as well as home health care recipients, were interviewed to determine their levels of emotional well-being and life satisfaction. Those living in the SNF's reported themselves to be the most satisfied with their living conditions and had the highest emotional health. A possible explanation for this finding is that all of the patients' needs—physical, emotional, social, and recreational—were taken care of in one place, where they were familiar with the routine.

While there continue to be reports of patient abuse, nursing home residents generally receive the needed levels of care. What may be missing, however, is the sense of belonging to an extended, caring family.

The Placement Decision. When a decision has been made for institutionalization, and when an SNF is seen as the appropriate placement, it is important to make the right choice of a facility. To do that requires a basic understanding of nursing homes and the emotional factors that go along with a placement decision. All nursing homes provide essentially the same levels of medical care and related services.

Public nursing homes are operated directly by the state or municipal government. They generally have the most beds per facility but make up only 10 percent of the SNF's in the United States. Only those individuals the government is directly responsible for are treated in these facilities. These usually include medically indigent or Medicaid-eligible people.

Voluntary facilities are operated by nonprofit organizations such as religious groups or fraternal orders. These types of facilities make up roughly 15 percent of nursing homes. The remaining facilities, 75 percent of the total, are smaller, proprietary facilities. They are privately owned and are operated for a profit. Both voluntary and proprietary SNF's serve both public and private patients (Murray & Glassberg, 1975).

Before considering placement in a nursing home, it is important to be sure that the patient is an appropriate candidate for an SNF. It has been estimated that as many as 40 percent of the patients in SNF's would do better in facilities giving lower levels of care (Reiff, 1980). Patients wind up in the SNF's because of a lack of other programs and poor reimbursement for home care. An additional reason is poor screening or use of inappropriate assessment tools (Salamon, 1984c). Most assessment forms are not completely objective measures and have questionable reliability (Kane & Kane, 1981).

Relocation is difficult for everyone, regardless of their age. Adjustment to an SNF, however, is especially difficult for older adults. It is associated with a loss of independence and freedom, separation from friends and important personal possessions, and, most significantly, loss of control over one's life. Easing the trauma of relocation requires finding the right facility with the proper programs and a caring staff.

For individuals who value religious observances, the nursing home should have a chapel with regular services. Patients who, for example, have eaten kosher foods all of their lives should not be forced to change their eating habits upon entering an SNF, so one that caters to this need should be found.

By allowing patients to bring along a few personal possessions, nursing homes help to preserve their patients' sense of dignity and keep them in touch with their past. Facilities that offer a wide variety of recreational programs should be selected, allowing residents to find the activities of most interest to them. There also should be an active resident council and the opportunity to pursue individual hobbies. Meals should be served in a sociable and pleasant surrounding, encouraging interaction and facilitating acceptance into the home's community. It also goes without saying that adequate health care services and proper staff–patient ratios be provided. The home also should have a clean appearance and should have only a mild disinfectant odor, if at all.

When families have to make the decision for placement, they usually do so with a sense of guilt and trepidation. Families may realize the need for institutionalization but may feel guilt at not being able to do more for the older adult family member. They may be fearful that their older parent or relative will not receive the right type of care. To help overcome these feelings, it is important for the family to visit a variety of facilities, if that is possible (Silverstone & Hyman, 1976). They should look for a facility that has the types of services just discussed.

It is also important, whenever possible, to have the patient visit the facilities personally and join in the selection process. In fact, it is an abuse of a person's humanity to exclude her or him from the decision-making process, provided of course that the person is competent to do so.

INNOVATIVE PROGRAMS

A variety of alternative health care programs for the elderly are presently being explored. Some of these projects are relatively new. Others are older, based on foreign models or models of care for other age groups, and still others are new only because of the creative approach used. In this last category is the use of SNF facilities to provide other services to nonresidents. In some demonstration projects, for example, older-adult daycare units are provided at nursing homes. In a more innovative approach, health care for frail elderly is combined with daycare for young children. Some nursing homes have onsite nurseries, allowing for enhanced intergenerational programming.

The Financial Question

One question still being debated is whether, despite the great expense involved in caring for individuals in a facility, alternative care programs are more cost effective than institutions. When the cost of rent, food, and caretaker time is taken into account, facility-based care may be less expensive than care provided in the home. There is still, however, an unquestioned conviction that anything that keeps the elderly out of institutions is desirable (Lashof, 1977).

As we have seen, both Medicaid and Medicare are structured to encourage institutionalization and are opposed to home health care. Suggestions for offsetting the inducement of institutionalization offered by Medicare and Medicaid range from changing the reimbursement structure to allowing federal and state tax deductions for families who provide home health care to their aging relatives. As we have seen, the Medicare statute specifically prohibits payment for services otherwise covered, if they are provided by members of one's household or family. Medicare currently pays for only limited home health care and does so only on a temporary basis. Homemaker services or help with activities of daily living are not reimbursed under Medicare.

In order to receive reimbursement for home health care services under Medicaid, all states now require a so called "spend down." Because Medicaid was designed for the medically indigent elderly, there is a ceiling on allowable income. If the frail older adult has more in financial resources than allowed, they cannot receive Medicaid benefits. Older individuals are therefore forced to give up, or "spend down," their assets in order to become eligible for these Medicaid benefits. Moreover, there are restrictions to the spend-down requirements. In instances where it is found that the elderly have disposed of assets within a recent period of time, they have the liability of paying for their care up to the amount spent down. These spend-down requirements also favor institutional care, for spending down occurs more rapidly when basic living needs, rather than being given at home, are provided in facilities where they can be considered as legitimate medical costs.

There have been proposals to alter these requirements. Suggestions include mandating that employers include certain long-term care benefits as part of their health insurance plans. These benefits would include not only the costs of institutional-based care but home health care as well. One suggested method of convincing private health care insurers to provide these services is by having portions of it underwritten by the federal government.

Another means of encouraging home health care is to allow individuals to claim a tax deduction when they contribute to the cost of health services for a family member who is not a member of the immediate household. This would encourage families to contribute to the sharing of home health care costs (Packwood, 1981).

There are, of course, situations where families cannot care for frail, elderly members at home. In addition to the financial responsibility and work needs of family members, the children of these elderly may themselves be old and in need of care. Older adults in their eighties often have children who are in their sixties. Even so, institutionalization may not be the only course of action.

Enriched Housing

One program designed to offer an alternative to institutionalization for the frail elderly who can no longer live on their own is enriched housing. These programs consist of shared group living arrangements where a number of older adults live together and are provided with the supportive services they need in order to maintain themselves in their own communities. These services include assistance in housekeeping, shopping, meal preparation, and personal care, and an around-the-clock, on-call emergency coverage program. The program is designed to maximize the residents' autonomy, independence, and sense of privacy. These innovative arrangements may be located within ordinary, publicly subsidized or private housing. Enriched housing programs are often located in buildings that also house the well elderly.

There are various models within the enriched housing concept. In one model, one large apartment with many bedrooms is shared. Each bedroom is a private residence for the individual client. Another approach is individual dwelling units. Small apartments or studios, each with only one resident, are provided in close proximity to other such units.

In most instances, there are limitations as to the number of units that may be devoted to enriched housing in any one building. This is done in order to preserve the noninstitutional atmosphere of the program.

Participation in enriched housing programs is usually limited to older adults who have a degree of functional impairment that would preclude independent living, yet the level of impairment may not be so severe as to require continuous nursing or medical supervision or full-time assistance with skills of daily living. In New York State for example, low-income residents of enriched housing who are eligible receive a state supplement above the federal Supplemental Security Income benefit. Until recently, this state benefit had been available to the impaired elderly only if they had been institutionalized.

A major aspect of the enriched housing approach is the emphasis placed on independence, within functional limits. Residents of such programs have their own rooms or apartments, share companionship with peers, and are provided for without the stigma of institutionalization.

Daycare Services

There are currently more than 600 programs in the United States offering daycare services for older adults (Ohnsorg, 1981). These services, variously titled *day treatment*, *day hospital*, and *day health care*, provide a variety of programs that offer support to frail, elderly community residents. Without such support these individuals would almost surely require full-time residence in a facility.

Daycare programs can be found in a variety of settings. They often are affiliated with medical institutions and may be on site at a hospital or nursing home. They also often are located in community centers and senior citizen centers.

There are three general goals for adult day care:

1. Rehabilitation for persons whose physical and social skills can be improved
2. Maintenance of current levels of functioning to slow or delay the deteriorative process
3. The provision of respite for those individuals who normally would care for the client in a home setting

The general requirements for admission to a day program are that the individuals (1) are considered medically at risk and (2) without the benefit of daycare would require institutionalization. Daycare programs offer medical, nursing, rehabilitation, nutritional, psychiatric, and social services to their clients. In addition, the daycare program offers planned social and recreational activities designed to prevent deterioration and enhance social interaction.

In California, a study of costs of providing adult daycare indicates that over $600 per month is spent on nursing home services under the Medical Program, California's Medicaid. Similar services when provided at an adult daycare program are only $450 per month (U.S. Senate, 1982).

Daycare programs are generally open Monday to Friday from 8:30 A.M. to 4:30 P.M. Some of the clients attend on a daily basis. Others attend only one or two days per week. The number of days in attendance is based on the client's need for care and the other services available to the client outside of the program. Some programs provide transportation, both picking up clients and taking them home at the end of the day. Daycare programs offer the opportunity to provide a comprehensive variety of programs to frail elderly, all in one environment. This eliminates the piecemeal aspect of care often seen in home care, and it also encourages socialization with peers.

Respite Care

Respite care, or temporary hospital care, is a program that began in England. The initial concept was to provide an institutional facility offering the same services found in skilled nursing facilities, for the same type of low-functioning, frail patient. The one major difference is the temporary nature of the institutionalization. Patients are brought to the facility and can remain in the institution for only a limited time. The amount of time spent in the facility is usually negotiated between the service provider at home, generally a family member, and the facility. There are often times when these family members, providing and supervising care for frail, ill, older adults, need some temporary relief from the responsibility. Perhaps they themselves become ill, or other family responsibilities arise, or they simply want to take a vacation. The caregiver negotiates the amount of time necessary for respite, during which time the ill family member is cared for by professionals in an institutional setting. This program offers an important alternative in preventing burnout by the family care providers.

Respite programs currently are being undertaken in the United States as demonstration projects with special grant funds. In order for such temporary care programs to become successful, reimbursement regulations may need some revision, to allow for changing the sites where care is offered.

Geriatric Foster Care

One of the least restrictive alternatives to institutional care for the elderly is geriatric foster care (Steinhauer, 1982). This program uses private family residences for the care of elderly persons who are not related to the homeowners.

There does not presently exist one particular model of geriatric foster care. The types of programs that offer foster care vary from state to state. Despite the current piecemeal nature of these programs, there is a general consensus that geriatric foster care should reach those older individuals whose functional and emotional status could best be served in a protective living arrangement. One approach is to match the needs of the older adult client with the provider's ability to attend to that need. Here, too, in order for such programs to become successful, reimbursement for care provided in the home should be made available as an alternative to institutionalization.

Echo Housing

One program that offers an alternative solution for a variety of both elderly and community problems is Elder Cottage Housing Opportunities, or ECHO housing (Hare, 1982).

Two major issues face us in terms of the housing needs of our society. One problem relates to the difficulty faced by young people in finding homes they can afford and that are not too large for their needs. Single-family zoning has produced neighborhoods of one-family homes to respond to the needs of the baby boom of the 1950s. These homes, however, no longer contain large families. The children have grown up and moved away, and the homes are too expensive for younger people to purchase, given the present economic environment. As a result of this historical event, we are confronted by the second issue: How can older adults utilize the extra space they now have in their large homes?

ECHO housing, or accessory apartments, provides a possible solution to both of these dilemmas. Based on the Australian concept of "granny flats," these apartments are designed as small, temporary living units that offer independent living for an older person while being contained within a larger home, thus, both the older homeowners and younger household can reside in the same house.

An important benefit of ECHO housing is the opportunity it presents for an exchange of income and services. Stronger, more able people can mow the lawn and take out the garbage. In return, the older adult can offer babysitting services or assist with other home chores. The overall benefits include making housing available to younger householders, while older householders maintain their own home and independent existence.

One major drawback to such programs is a legal issue. Most neighborhoods are zoned for single-unit housing only and do not allow alternatives such as accessory apartments. Currently, only the state of Pennsylvania and the towns of Weston, Connecticut, Portland, Oregon, and Babylon, New York have legalized such housing alternatives.

Emergency Response Systems

The variety of electronic devices and computer applications invented almost daily have expanded the possibilities for providing more efficient home health care alternatives for the frail elderly. As mentioned previously, home monitoring services currently exist. These programs automatically dial a central monitoring station when activated by a community resident. The notification indicates that the individual is in need of assistance, and the central station dispatches help.

Other possible future alternatives include monitoring heart rate, body temperature, and other bodily functions, via the telephone. Computers linked from individuals' homes to central medical stations could do the monitoring and recommend care options, such as changes in diet.

The future of innovative concepts is unlimited; however, innovation and new alternatives to long-term care should not be substituted for attempts at improving institutional services for those who have no other choice (Kane & Kane, 1980). What also requires careful attention is the way in which new approaches are performed. They should be applied in a humane and caring fashion in a way that offers not only medical care but social and emotional comfort, along with human contact and warmth.

HOSPICES AND THE TERMINALLY ILL

There is a dearth of essential literature on management techniques for dealing with the multiple needs of terminally ill and for helping with the feelings that arise when professionals deal with these patients (Kalish, 1978). Kübler-Ross (1969) proposes that dying patients progress through a series of five emotional stages prior to death. During the first two stages, terminally ill people *deny* the impending death and become *angry* at the prospect of death. Then they alternately *bargain* with a higher power to spare them and become *depressed*. These feelings can be coupled with a pervasive sense of hopelessness and may interfere with the delivery of needed health care (Abramson et al., 1981). The fifth stage is the period during which the dying individual begins to *accept* their fate. Others have found that, despite the overpowering sense of loss, there is no uniform coping pattern (Goleman, 1982).

Antagonistic relationships also may develop between the health care provider and the family of a dying person. Doctors, particularly specialists, offer their services in the impersonal hospital or nursing home setting, rarely spending sufficient time relating to the needs of the patient, let alone the patient's family. Though health care providers must deal with it regularly, there is still a fear of death and a sense of failure when a patient dies. Doctors are being admonished to provide comfort from pain and a sense of attention to their terminally ill patients (Buckingham, 1979).

It has been suggested that individuals who are terminally ill might be more comfortable at home in their few remaining days. There is a good deal of benefit that people may gain from the familiar environment of their own home. Caring for a terminally ill individual in their remaining days at home also may offer the family an opportunity to confront and accept the reality of the situation.

In instances where it is impossible for the dying patients to receive terminal care in their own homes, a movement that began in the United States in the early 1970s may offer a reasonable alternative. The hospice movement is based on the well-known St. Christopher's Hospice outside of London. Hospices are institutions that specialize in the care of terminally ill patients. They are usually small facilities with no more than about 50 beds, often with as few as 15. Some hospices are integrated into hospitals or other facilities. The goal of the hospice movement is to allow terminally ill patients to live their remaining days in dignity. While there are no exact figures, the majority of those who use hospices are older adults.

The type of care offered by hospices is palliative. There is no attempt made to cure the illness or to use heroic efforts to extend life. The emphasis is placed on relief of pain and providing emotional support, not only for the ill individual but for the family as well.

The schedules of care in the hospice are based on the patients' desires and not the institution's needs. Meals are served when the patient is hungry and often include alcoholic beverages. Large doses of pain-killing medications may be administered, at the patient's own request.

An important component of hospice care is the involvement of family and community. Because the death of a family member affects the entire family, hospices treat not just the dying individual but the person's family as well. The informal family care providers are encouraged to continue to assist in providing care, even when the patient is in the hospice. In addition, a good many hospices rely quite heavily on community volunteers to assist in the provision of services. This integration of formal and informal care providers make the hospice a unique service organization.

There has been some opposition voiced toward the hospice movement. Some physicians see it as an abandonment of hope. Refusing to treat terminally ill patients, they say, is an insult to the medical profession. Another fear is that hospices will be opened by unscrupulous individuals interested only in profit making. Indeed, it has been estimated that as many as 25 hospices opened each month in 1982. Others respond that hospices provide good medical care when little remains to be done (Newsline, 1979).

Hospice care is currently covered under Medicare only as a brief demonstration project. There are bills, though, before both houses of Congress to provide for reimbursement for physician's services, homemaker services, drug therapy, and counseling when these are provided in a hospice.

Terminally ill people have a number of concerns beyond the immediate care they are receiving. Funerals are an important consideration for ill older adults, who often hold deep religious values. They are interested in knowing where their remains will be buried, and occasionally they want some involvement in preparing for the funeral itself. Often burial sites and caskets are purchased in advance. When this is not the case, it is important to aid the family in avoiding unscrupulous funeral chapels.

Other concerns of terminally ill elderly include legal issues, such as the disposition of the estate and will. They need to make sure that it is accurate and up to date, in order to feel as if things are in order before they depart.

Those who work with the terminally ill may find it hard to deal with the individual as a whole person. Professionals sometimes may refer to the "cancer case in room 620," or use some similar distancing language. It is imperative, though, to remember that all patients, even dying patients, are whole human beings, with feelings and needs of their own that should be heard and acted upon.

Another defense mechanism used by professionals when dealing with the terminally ill is false happiness. While being forever somber is not appropriate, neither is a false sense of gaiety. Patients should be treated as real people, with real emotions, who need to both cry and laugh, argue and express a full range of emotions, and need to be responded to honestly.

Workers also have to help comfort the family of the dead or dying individual. Here too, a sense of warmth, comfort, and concern is generally the best approach.

SUMMARY

We have reviewed the variety of health care and related programs older adults generally have available to them. There is a continuum of care that corresponds to level of illness and ranges from health-education and recreation programs to home care options and skilled nursing facilities. Some new and innovative programs designed to maintain older adults in their own communities were described. Just as important as physical health are the mental health needs of the elderly. The next chapter examines psychological health and illness.

3

Mental Health Needs

PERSONALITY AND DEVELOPMENT

It has become common knowledge that an individual's personality and choice of lifestyle can predispose that person to certain illnesses and even death (Engel, 1971; Schmale, 1972). For instance, smoking has been shown to cause lung cancer and heart disease. In the case of heart disease, the ways in which people respond to their environment may determine the possibility of their getting a heart attack (Friedman & Rosenman, 1974).

A relationship may have been found between personality and long-term well-being. A study performed at the Institute of Human Development at the University of California in Berkely (Eichorn, Clausen, Haan, Honzik & Mussen, 1981) seems to have found some of the essential threads of personality development. By interviewing and testing the same people and their children for the past 40 years, these researchers feel that they have found the "building blocks of a well-integrated personality." Among their findings, they point out that those people who are emotionally and psychologically stable at the age of 30 will more than likely remain that way into their seventies. The reverse is also true. Young adults who are depressed, fearful, rigid, and report themselves to be sickly are still troubled in life's later years. Somewhat similar results indicating the stability of personality traits throughout adulthood were found in other studies (Costa & McCrae, 1980).

Developmental Changes

When one studies the entire human lifespan from birth to death, certain significant shifts in motivation, needs, frustrations, and problems become noticeable. Several researchers have documented the more frequently occurring shifts (Haan, 1977; Vaillant, 1977).

Frenkel-Brunswik Psychological Growth Curve. In a pioneering study performed in Austria in 1933 (Frenkel-Brunswik, 1968), it was found that there are five major phases of psychological development in the human lifespan. These phases form a psychological growth curve that partially parallels what used to be thought of as the average human biological growth curve (see Figure 3–1).

The biological growth curve consists of three stages. In the first stage, the stage of *progressive growth*, the organism is maturing biologically to the limits of its development. This stage lasts until the age of roughly 25. The second stage, *stability of growth*, lasts until the age of roughly 45, until the final stage, the *period of decline* is reached. Biologically, all systems begin to decline in their ability to function at optimum levels during the second stage.

The concept of a biological growth curve has been shown to be less useful as overall health care has improved. The period of stability has become increasingly extended, and the period of decline dramatically shortened (Fries, 1983). Nevertheless, the major developmental theories still assume that the curve exists and that psychological development parallels it.

The first of the five developmental/psychological periods of life, according to Frenkel-Brunswik (1968) is one in which the child lives at home and has only narrow outside social interest. The second stage begins in adolescence and is marked by the first steps taken toward independence in activities and social relations. The third stage begins somewhere around the twenty-eighth birthday. It lasts until about age 50 and includes the largest number of dimensions. This period corresponds to the biological curve as being the most stable and productive period of life. The person in this stage has the most outside interests.

The fourth period, as in the biological curve, is measured by the amount of regression or withdrawal from outside activities. The researchers suggested that this period is fraught with both psychological and biological crises. The fifth phase begins at about age 65 and sharply accentuates the decline noted in the previous stage, which is marked by sickness and death of loved ones. People in this stage become self-centered and lose almost all of their outside interests.

This study was performed early in this century, before many of the major advances of medicine were made which led to the increased life expectancy we now experience. The older individuals in that study

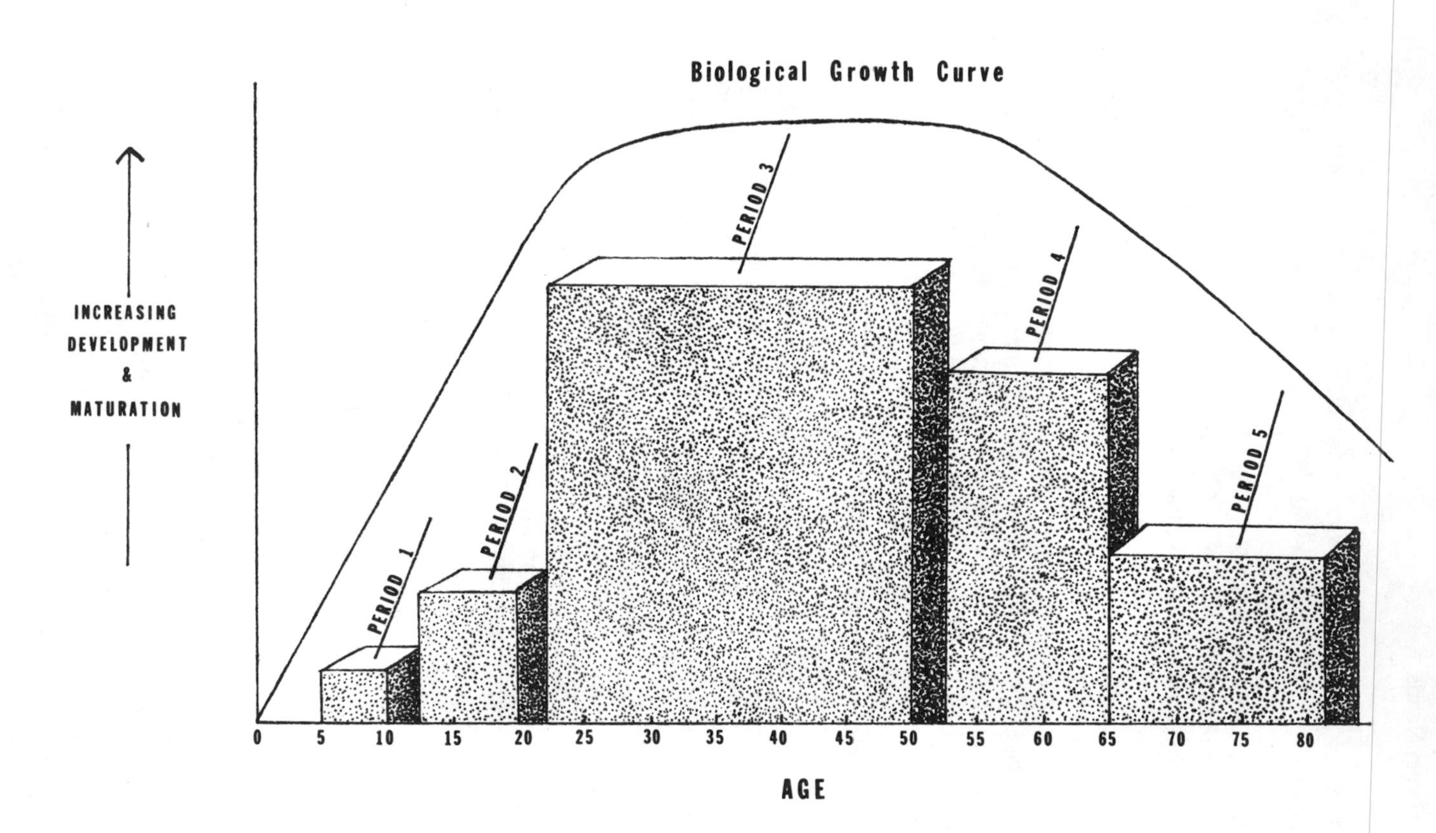

Figure 3–1 The biological growth curve and Frenkel-Brunswik's (1968) psychological development periods.

may have been too preoccupied with the stressful biological changes of aging to have answered in a more positive manner. Currently, due to the increased and improved medical care available, one finds that older people not only do not give up their outside interests but in certain instances look for new, productive hobbies and interests.

Eriksonian Theory. Somewhat parallel and yet contrasting to the preceding study is Erikson's (1950) developmental theory. Erikson hypothesized that life can always be developing in a positive way. Eight stages of ego development from infancy to old age are theorized. In each stage, the ego or self may face a crisis, and it may grow positively or it may decline.

According to Erikson, the first stage of life is marked by the conflict of basic trust versus mistrust. In this period the child either learns to trust its caregivers and eventually the greater social network or develops a deep sense of mistrust.

The next stage is the period referred to as the time of autonomy versus shame and doubt. Here the child learns to develop a sense of control over itself or, negatively, experiences a sense of pervasive doubt.

When the child begins to explore its world it faces the developmental crisis of initiative versus guilt. Either the child is rewarded for taking the initiative of learning about the environment or is scolded, and hence forms an underlying sense of guilt.

At about the time a child enters school the conflict of industry versus inferiority develops. The child will either learn to work at a task that will be rewarded or will feel a sense of inferiority for not performing up to a standard.

During adolescence, the conflict revolves around identity: having a sense of one's general road or career path versus a feeling of role confusion.

In the sixth stage, the period of young adulthood, the developmental conflict centers on intimacy versus social isolation. It is during this stage that individuals form lasting relationships with others or choose to live lives of isolation.

Stages seven and eight are of primary interest in our study of older adults. The seventh stage, the age of middle adulthood, is marked by the development of *generativity,* that is, an expansion of interests with a concurrent sense of having contributed to the future. If this does not occur, then what takes its place is *ego stagnation,* Erikson's term for the negative potential of this period.

Late adulthood is the period for the eighth stage, which is marked by a struggle between *ego integrity* and a *sense of despair*, in Erikson's terms. Either one accepts one's life as having been productive, meaningful, and successful or one spends one's final days dejected and living in fear of inevitable death.

Role Theories. There are three classical theories in the gerontological literature, regarding optimum patterns of aging: activity theory, disengagement theory, and continuity theory. They are based on the observations that as people grow older their styles of living and roles in life change. These theories are often invoked when discussing the personality patterns of the aged.

The first view, *activity theory*, assumes that, excepting the inevitable biological decline, older people are the same as middle-aged individuals. They have the same basic biological and psychological needs. Their decline, however, results in society's withdrawal from the aged person. The successful aged individuals are those who, through their own roles in life, are able to maintain activity successfully by resisting the dwindling social group available to them (Palmore, 1979). Many have concluded that maintaining an active role in old age is a positive predictor of well-being (Larson, 1978; Markides & Martin, 1979; Riley & Foner, 1968).

Disengagement theory (Cumming & Henry, 1961) is often viewed as a mutual agreement struck upon by the aged and society. Both withdraw from each another. The aged person accepts this psychological distance and uses it to invest more time in personal needs. This theory assumes that older people should acquiesce naturally to a lower state of activity, in keeping with their lessened abilities. Disengagement theory suggests that the aged withdraw from society for their own sense of emotional well-being. There has been little evidence indicating that this theory is highly accurate.

In fact, observation shows that neither theory can be universally applied. Aging individuals may or may not disengage from their middle-life activities, and they may or may not slow down in their social activities (Salamon, 1985b). Most obviously, however, is the simple fact that aged individuals can never completely separate from a society whose values they have spent a whole life internalizing, no matter how much the society may have changed. Also, as has been noted, personality patterns may be somewhat stable over an individual's life (Holzberg, 1982). The *theory of continuity* (Covey, 1982) therefore suggests that, as individuals age their habits, preferences, and commitments become more discernible (Neugarten, 1977). Older people's roles can be explained best only by examining their lifelong response patterns (Atchley, 1972). Those individuals who lived their lives in solitude will continue in that manner, while those who were active and outgoing will continue to be that way.

Personality Types and Mental Illness

In an early attempt to explore the relationship between personality and mental disorder in older adults, Lowenthal (1965) analyzed data from a large group of older people who had been hospitalized for mental illness. What she found was that mental illness and social isolation seem to go hand in hand in the aged. In old age, mental illness may be the cause of isolation, but the reverse also may be true: Isolation may be linked with developing a mental illness. Bennett (1980) also concluded that isolation can result in the development of behavior patterns that are associated with a mental disorder.

There have been several studies that have examined how people with different personality types, particularly the aged, cope with emotional stresses. Butler (1963) found that personality often dictates how one responds to the crises of old age. If the individual has always had a well-developed personality, including a strong use of insight allowing accurate perceptions of the changed circumstances of old age, reaction to stress will be healthier than in an individual with a negative outlook on life.

Another interesting finding is that some personality traits thought to be maladaptive at younger ages are thought to be adaptive in the later ones. Denial of aging was one of these traits. If the aging individual is capable of maintaining a sense of identity in the face of societal pressures and biases against the aging process, that person may be said to be denying aging. At the same time, the person is exhibiting a pattern of development that may be adaptive. The older person, by the strength of her or his personality, refuses to take on the social role of the sickly older person.

In a similar view, an informal study of 80 people between the ages of 70 and 90 found that those older adults who imagined themselves to be younger than they actually were, looked, dressed, acted, and spoke as if they were younger (Salamon, 1984b). Results of a long-term study of personality also bear this out (Granick & Patterson, 1971). In this study it was found that the response of healthy older adults to personality assessment tests were very similar to those of younger adults.

Personality Changes

There are a number of personality changes that have been found to occur as people get very old and closer to death. Two of the most important of these are life review and terminal drop.

Life Review. Butler (1963) found that most of the aged like to reminisce, reviewing the many experiences of their lives. He called this process the *life review*. Butler noted the possibility of a good many, varied behavioral and affective states that can result from the life review, ranging from mild depressions to feelings of anxiety, guilt, and constant obsessional rumination. Rather than finding heightened self-awareness in those individuals near death, one can easily find increasing rigidity (Butler, 1975). This may result from their feeling that they have not accomplished their life's goals.

There has been an indication, though, that reminiscing is not only useful and natural but a productive mental activity in the elderly. Ebersole (1976) observed that the most well-adjusted of her elderly patients were those who were able to review the "good old days."

Terminal Drop. It has been suggested by several researchers that as death draws nearer there is an unexplained, sometimes sudden drop in psychological and intellectual functioning among old people. Lieberman (1965) reviewed several studies that found that psychological changes can occur several months prior to an older adult's death. Another study (Riegel & Riegel, 1972) found that psychological changes can take place up to five years prior to death. In still another study, researchers found that older adults were more accurate in predicting their own death than were their physicians (Botwinick, West, & Storandt, 1978).

This information may be important for health care providers, for, if they are alert and recognize these changes, it may help them to deal better with possible difficulties or prepare their patient for death.

Summary

To summarize, it has been shown that, in general,

1. People who have healthy personalities will maintain healthy personalities as they age.
2. People with maladaptive personalities may have a harder time coping with their own aging.
3. Denial of one's own aging may be healthy.

4. Social isolation may be linked with developing a mental illness.
5. Reminiscence, or the life review, is a normal process for those near to death.
6. Unexplained changes that occur in older adults' intellectual or psychological functioning may be predictive of impending death.

SOCIOECONOMIC FACTORS IN MENTAL HEALTH

It is an accepted fact that depression may be caused by loss. In this sense, it is analogous to the life state of the aged, whose socioeconomic environments are often characterized by losses so great that personality alone may not be a sufficient tool for coping.

It has been shown that an individual's behavior varies directly with the characteristics of the immediate socioeconomic environment. If you ask any person who he or she really is, the most common response would be that person's work or occupational status. People also are judged by their social contacts and the neighborhood in which they live. It is in these three areas—work, social contacts, and living arrangements—that the aged suffer the most anxiety, because it is in these areas that their status is radically changed.

Retirement

Our society, built on the Protestant ethic of hard work and just rewards, has a built-in paradox: retirement. This is the time when a worker is expected to stop working and lead a life of leisure. Several difficulties often occur among those who retire. First of all, income generally decreases after retirement. Census figures bear out the dramatic effect retirement has on income by showing that many people become poor for the first time in their lives only after they retire (U.S. Bureau of the Census, 1982b).

Retirement, however, is not just an economic event. It is also a social event with far-ranging implications. Work can equal the level of self-esteem an individual experiences. Work, or an activity that is equally as meaningful to the individual, appears to be an essential component in the maintenance of mental health. Yet, regardless of congressional legislation, the median age for retirement is steadily dropping (U.S. Senate, 1982).

There is a further problem particular to our advanced society. As the general health of society is improved, the size of its available labor force is increased. At the same time, also as a consequence of technological advances, automation in industry is reducing the demand for labor. While the children of the 1950s baby boom have all grown up and entered the work force, there still exists the fiscal and philosophical problem of finding jobs for all those who want to work. One way of controling that problem is through retirement (Bradford Healthfield Newsletter, 1979).

Monk (1975) reported that many men look upon retirement as an end that would bring rejection, lack of recognition, and death. The men he interviewed felt that life without work had no meaning. The predominant feeling was that death was the only way to retire from life. On the other hand, for those elderly who can financially afford to retire, there is a conflict between the historical convictions of the work ethic and contemporary ways that include retirement resorts or villages. Thus, based upon an individual's expectations, some workers may look upon retirement as a new role to be viewed with a heightened sense of positive anticipation.

Even those who accept the retirement village lifestyle at the outset may be forced later to reconsider. There are a great many researchers who point to the negative aspects of isolating age groups (Daum, 1982; Donahue, Thompson, & Curren, 1977). While peer support is extremely important, it cannot make up for the fact that isolation by age, as happens in a retirement village, may be viewed by some as no better than placement in an asylum. Kübler-Ross (1975) noted that, even though we may give our older adults "color television . . ., swimming pools, golf courses and dancing facilities . . ., we deprive them of the chance to still serve. Living means to give and to take . . . and to serve others—and it is the latter that is often missing in our retirement centers . . ., which [may] result in the wish to die, because life isn't worth living anymore" (p. 19).

A review of some of the changes that may result from retirement is in order. They are

1. A significant decrease in income
2. A possible loss of self-esteem
3. A sense of rejection at not being an actively contributing worker
4. Resulting isolation

While losing a job is a potentially stressful event at any age, the level of stress tolerance in the aged is weakened, thus making it a more difficult situation to cope with. In addition, discrimination due to age for those who wish to continue working is also a stab at one's sense of self-esteem. Congress has all but outlawed mandatory retirement before age 70. While this is an important act, this law has severe drawbacks. To bypass the law several companies offer financial inducements for early retirement. The immediate payoff is attractive; however, the long-term benefits are doubtful. Another drawback in the law is that it suggests that discrimination continues to be okay in relation to the very old.

Recognizing that the key to a successful retirement is making the retiree feel needed (Horn, 1975), several organizations have established preretirement counseling programs. These courses help those about to retire to understand what they will be facing. Groups meet to discuss some of the family problems experienced with retirement, and the greatest stress is placed on the creative use of leisure time so that it is seen as productive (O'Meara, 1977).

There are those, however, who do not wish to retire but would rather continue working. For some, taking positions as volunteers in hospitals, nursing homes, or schools provides a sense of self-esteem and removes the feelings of isolation. Others may try to band together to form job-seekers' groups that act as both personnel agencies and support groups for those older adults who are seeking employment (Gray, 1983).

Social Contacts

The loss of social contacts is another important factor affecting the aged. Depression can be caused by the loss of loved ones or those with whom one regularly socialized.

Loss of Spouse. The loss of a loved one can be so stressful that it has been shown to be related to higher death rates, particularly for males (Rowland, 1977). Hendin (1973) found that physical complaints such as arthritis and chest pains increased following the loss of a loved one. Hendin also reported that bereavement can be so stressful for both widows and widowers that they are more likely to die in the year immediately after the loss of a spouse than married people matched for age and social class.

The Family. It had been assumed for many years that as people aged their families withdrew from them, creating even more intense isolation. Happily this has been shown not to be the case. When family networks exist for the elderly, which is most often the case, there is usually a reasonable amount of contact (Brody, Davis, Fulcomer, & Johnson, 1979; Shanas, 1979).

The Social Network. Though family members may continue to maintain strong social ties, the number of friends available to older adults dwindles as a result of relocation and death. As this occurs it becomes more difficult for the older adult to maintain social ties. In extreme cases this can lead to isolation (Rathbone-McCuan & Hashimi, 1982), which can lead to depression and other symptoms of mental disorder.

Living Arrangements

The living arrangements of the elderly may be another contributing factor in the development of mood disturbances. In our society what is commonly found is that the aged tend to remain in the older, poorer, and more dangerous communities. A survey of over 300 older adults, performed in the New York City area (Nev, 1976), indicated that the aged remained in poorer neighborhoods even when other accommodations were available in better areas. They did so for two reasons: (1) familiarity with surroundings and (2) fear of the unknown. These individuals appeared to be locked into a depression of their own making. They feared leaving their own apartments, yet they insisted that it was no better elsewhere, without truly knowing.

There has been a long-standing debate as to whether or not relocation, or moving from one living environment to another, results in excessive stress. *Relocation trauma* or *transfer trauma,* as it is often referred to, is said to be a result of loss of social and environmental familiarity (Lawton & Nahemow, 1973). Presently, however, there is no clear evidence indicating that moving from one living environment to another, in and of itself, causes excessive stress (Borup, 1982).

AFFECTIVE DISORDERS

Symptomology

Before examining the techniques of intervention, a review of the basic aspects of affective disorders or depression is called for. The signs and symptoms of depression, considered to be a disturbance of mood, include

1. Continual sad mood; the person is always melancholic
2. Self-deprecating thoughts; comments such as, "I am useless"
3. Feelings of inability to cope
4. Feelings of hopelessness and helplessness

5. Marked loss of interest in work or activities
6. Agitated behavior
7. Anxiety
8. Vegetative signs, including loss of appetite and insomnia
9. Suicidal thoughts, often verbalized
10. Particularly in the elderly, heightened physical complaints such as chest pains or digestive tract complaints (Mendels, 1970)

Berezin (1972) summed up depressions in the elderly by saying, "Depression contains a quality of hopelessness in the face of events one would like to control but cannot" (p. 220).

An interesting note is that many of the symptoms of depression are also shared by those suffering from senile dementia. The problems of differentiating between depression and dementia will be taken up in greater detail in a later section. At this point it is appropriate to say that an incorrect diagnosis of dementia, rather than depression, can lead to even worse depression.

Etiology

There are many theories regarding the causes of affective disorders. Depressions are sometimes seen as a form of guilt turned inward. Certain behavioral concepts attribute depression to the loss of a positive reinforcer. There are several biochemical and genetic hypotheses too. Among them is the theory that low levels of brain catecholamines, norepinephrines in particular, are highly correlated with depression and may even be implicated as causal agents (Coppen, 1976). There is also evidence for a genetic predisposition to mood disturbances; that is, the children of depressed parents may be slightly more likely to get depressed than those whose parents did not have the disorder.

As of now, no one theory has been shown to be accurate in explaining the causes of depression. What is currently accepted as fact is that reactive depression can be brought on by the loss of a stable environment and loved ones. It is also known that depression in the aged is often based on loss of positive reinforcers (Eisdorfer & Lawton, 1973; Kernberg, 1977).

Suicide and death are related to extreme forms of depression in all age groups. Kraus and Lillienfield (1955) reported a higher incidence of mortality within the first year after the death of a loved one. Similarly, Sainsbury (1955) reported that, at advanced ages most suicides are committed by males who are suffering from depressive psychoses. He pointed out that the suicides are caused by illness, bereavement, and loneliness. Two important corollaries are that the rate of successful suicide attempts increases with age and the methods employed become more violent with age. As early as the mid nineteenth century, physicians had begun pointing out that in certain cases mild reactive depressions in old people could lead to suicide (Rosen, 1968). In fact, suicide is the eleventh leading cause of death for people between the ages of 65 and 74 (National Center for Health Statistics, 1983).

By definition, those who survive to be elderly are the most fit and are therefore called upon to experience more losses than any other age group. Those people currently over the age of 60 have already lived through three wars and a major economic depression. In addition, they are faced with having to see those whom they have loved pass on in ever increasing numbers. Their environment is continually changing. Imagine the change from a farming society, only beginning to become industrialized, to a society that has sent people to the moon and you only scratch the surface of change the present cohort of elderly have witnessed. They also feel themselves changing, and they may yearn for stability. If they cannot cope normally, in certain instances they cope abnormally. They may revert to depression and, if not caught in time, possibly suicide. The next three sections will examine the areas from which major daily changes emanate in the lives of the elderly.

BIOLOGICAL FACTORS IN MENTAL HEALTH

While personality and socioeconomic factors seem to affect individuals differently, biological factors tend to have a more universal aspect to them. There are some clear biological explanations for the sluggish responsiveness often seen in the elderly. With increasing age, there is a decrease in the excitability of the autonomic nervous system. The autonomic nervous system is that portion of the nervous system that is commonly referred to as the involuntary or automatic system because it is not under a person's immediate control. This system includes the mechanisms that mobilize the body during stress and also run the body under normal conditions. Included among these are organs such as the heart, lungs, and stomach. As the system gets older, response time gets slower.

Aside from the neurological changes, there are other more observable and readily measurable biological impairments associated with old age that are fairly universal. These changes can contribute to personality changes, disturbances of mood, and more severe psychological impairment. For example, hearing ability declines with age. Though this decline varies in degree from individual to individual, loss of hearing, or presbycusis, is a specific problem of the aged (Oyer & Oyer, 1979). The ability to hear sounds in the higher frequencies diminishes, and normal background noise tends to get confused with conversation. Thirty percent of all older people have a moderate to severe hearing loss. Ferguson (1976) points out the problems that confront the elderly who have a hearing deficit: "A person with a hearing problem frequently suffers from the lack of patience and understanding from those around him. Family and friends tend to avoid conversations, and the hearing-impaired person will most likely withdraw. . . . Social activities may be restricted, if not dropped altogether" (p. 11). Park and Shapiro (1976) note that deafness also contributes to paranoia, because people become suspicious as they misinterpret what they can hardly hear (Watts, 1980).

Other sensory changes take place in the aged. Visual changes often can be more debilitating than auditory changes. Inability to filter out glare is the most common visual deficit in the aged. Also, colors fade and depth perception weakens. Cataracts, which are due to a clouding of the lens and loss of fluid in the eyes, are a particular problem.

Because of changes in taste and smell and in the condition of gums and teeth, elderly people often do not eat as well as they should. There is a loss of fine muscle control, and ordinary degrees of hot and cold become difficult to distinguish. There is also a significant diminution of vital lung capacity with aging. Certain aspects of memory decline, specifically those related to making speedy responses. It is important to stress that this does not mean that normal aging results in a decline of intelligence. Quite the contrary; verbal ability continues to increase with age.

A decline in physical abilities may cause individuals to become less socially active. For example, older people who have to climb stairs to leave or return to their apartments may eventually find the task too demanding and so will stay home, isolated. Some physical changes can result in confusion, which then may be misdiagnosed as senility. Confusion also can also result from other common biological conditions, such as everyday infections of the respiratory or gastrointestinal tract, bone fractures, and surgery. These physical factors have this effect because older people, cast in the helpless role by society, are even more helpless when they feel the loss of bodily control and normal biological mechanisms. When a normally independent older person no longer can walk because of a bone fracture, depression and confusion can result, especially if the person is then further restricted by loss of social supports.

DEMENTIA

While many times confusion and disorientation may be due to social, environmental, or physical factors, it is also possible for these symptoms to result from organic changes in the brain, referred to as dementia (Brink, 1980). This can be caused by normal biological deterioration with age, with the result that intellectual functioning, in particular memory and orientation, become impaired. The terms *senile dementia* and *senility* are used to describe the loss of memory that occurs as people get older. Dementia can occur at any age, however, and can be caused by any number of diseases (Russel, 1981). The symptoms of dementia are

1. A loss of intellectual abilities sufficient to interfere with social functioning, but not involving delirium or loss of alertness or consciousness
2. Loss of memory, particularly short-term memory
3. Impaired judgment or impaired thought processes
4. Typically, but not always clear symptoms of depression

Dementias that are due exclusively to organic causes in the brain and most often linked with aging generally fall into one of two categories: multi-infract dementia and primary degenerative dementia (American Psychiatric Association, 1980).

Multi-infarct Dementia

Multi-infarct dementia is most typically a result of changes that take place in the blood vessels of the brain. It used to be assumed that the forgetfulness of aging was due to so-called "hardening of the arteries." While this has been shown not to be the case, multi-infarct dementia can occur when blood vessels in the brain become blocked or rupture.

Typically, when a person has a stroke, technically referred to as a *cerebrovascular accident* or CVA, a blood vessel in a particular portion of the brain malfunctions and as a result the oxygen carried in the blood does not get to the brain cells. When this happens the area of the brain fed by this blood vessel dies. When strokes are major and effect large portions of the brain, they can cause significant changes in the person, including loss of the ability to walk, talk, or feed themselves. As a general rule, though, a single stroke does not cause dementia. Multi-infarct dementia occurs when an individual experiences a series of ministrokes, each affecting different regions of the brain over a period of time, causing cumulative damage.

A person who has multi-infarct dementia will have other indications of vascular disease or disturbances in the circulatory system. There also may be a significant history of hypertension, and there will be neurological problems including weakness, difficulty in walking, and slowed or absent reflexes.

The course of this disease is usually erratic. It has a sudden onset, and, while deterioration proceeds in a stepwise fashion, its pace usually fluctuates. Early diagnosis of hypertension and vascular disease can help to curtail further deterioration.

Primary Degenerative Dementia

Unlike multi-infarct dementia, primary degenerative dementia (American Psychiatric Association, 1980) has a slow, gradual onset. While all the symptoms remain essentially the same, primary degenerative dementia often involves a wider range of intellectual deficits that get progressively worse over time. Often referred to as Alzheimer's disease or Senile Dementia of the Alzheimer's Type (SDAT), this dementia is caused not by changes in the blood vessels but by neurological problems in the brain. In one type, there is an accumulation of abnormal fibers that tangle and choke off the nerve cells of the brain. These fibers are called neurofibrillary tangles. The other change in brain cells that causes primary degenerative dementia is senile plaques. Throughout the brain, nerve endings deteriorate and block the transfer of information from one nerve cell to another.

While multi infarct dementia is not a very common disorder, Alzheimer's disease is. It is estimated that approximately 3 percent of those over the age of 65 have primary degenerative dementia, and the likelihood of getting the disease increases with age. It has been said that more people die with a diagnosis of Alzheimer's disease than the most common form of cancer, lung cancer (Terry, 1983).

The disease follows a slow, continual, deteriorative path, going through several stages (Reisberg et al., 1982):

1. *Early confusion.* Signs begin to emerge that the person is suffering from forgetfulness. She may have gotten lost on her way home from work, have difficulty finding words and names, begin to deny-

strenuously that there is a problem, and show signs of developing anxiety.

2. *Late confusion.* The individual becomes quite moody, using denial very frequently. There are clear signs of disorientation to place and possibly forgetfulness in regard to personal history.

3. *Early dementia.* The person needs help to survive; she cannot survive on her own. There is difficulty recognizing and recalling the names of some family members, and dressing can be performed but requires supervision.

4. *Middle dementia.* There are signs of being unaware of surroundings, and the person clearly is disoriented to time and place and occasionally to person. She may wander off and get lost; become agitated, particularly at nighttime; and is having increasing difficulty speaking.

5. *Late dementia.* The person becomes incontinent, disinterested in food, may lose the ability to walk, and often loses all verbal abilities.

The stage of middle dementia is the longest one in the disease, lasting as long as five to 10 years. The last stage, late dementia, is generally the briefest and lasts no more than two years. During all the stages, but particularly in the first three, individuals suffering from primary degenerative dementia show signs of depression, moodiness, and agitation.

Diagnosis of Dementia

A particular concern of the practicing gerontologist is to differentiate accurately between dementia and depression so that accurate interventions can be made. Until recently, it was not uncommon to find that, when older adults showed signs of forgetfulness, moodiness, and anxiety, they were wrongly diagnosed as suffering from dementia rather than depression (Salamon, 1979). Though clinical descriptions of Alzheimer's disease have been available for over 50 years, it is only within the last five years that the disease process has been described in detail (Reisberg, 1983). In this section we will review the different responses to assessment that individuals suffering from depression and dementia may make. Before that, however, it is important to examine another area of difficulty for older adults, one that may contribute to moodiness and forgetfulness.

Because of increased biological decline and subsequent susceptibility to illness, the aged take three times as many drugs as all other age groups combined (Hanan, 1978; Harper, 1984). Higher rates of medication use lead to more frequent adverse reactions and negative interactions between drugs. What is ironic is the fact that iatrogenically induced illness, which is illness that is caused by the treatment, often escapes detection because the symptoms also may mimic stereotyped behavior of old age. For example, drugs often perscribed for the treatment of fluid retention, diuretics, can cause symptoms of forgetfulness, confusion, weakness, anxiety, incontinence, anorexia, and tremor. The administration of antihistamines to the elderly can result in possible confusion and behavioral disturbances. Paradoxically, antidepressants also can cause behavioral confusion in the aged.

Biological Tests. As we have seen, the symptoms of organic mental disorders are common to functional depression, thus adding to the difficulty in establishing an accurate diagnosis. Because dementia is caused by deterioration in either the blood vessels or nerve cells in the brain, it is believed that diagnosis sometimes can be made by the use of x-rays of the brain. Several techniques have been devised for performing these x-rays. The most invasive type requires injecting a contrast medium—air or radio-opaque material—into the blood vessels in the head and taking radiographs of the brain. A popular new method is the CAT (Computerized Axial Tomography) scan, in which a computerized scanning machine produces three-dimensional pictures of cross-sections of the brain. Both methods have their drawbacks. The first can be painful and is likely to result in depressive responses. The second is relatively new, not widely used, and is highly expensive. Limited use can lead to questionable validity for comparison in a good many cases (Cutler et al., 1984).

An even newer method is Positron Emission Transaxial Tomography (PETT). A review of this system indicates that it is an improvement on the CAT scan, since the CAT scan gives only an anatomic view of brain structure, whereas the PETT offers a view of functioning within the brain. As it is currently constructed, the system's potential is of value primarily for the examination of patients receiving therapy for brain tumors. Its reliability for the detection of senile plaques has yet to be determined (McKhann et al., 1984).

Verbal Tests. As we have noted, the significant symptoms of the dementias are impairments in orientation, specifically time, place, and person. These impairments may be qualitatively or quantitatively different from the confusion and disorientation present in depression. What follows is a list of interview questions excerpted from a standard mental-status interview, plus the different responses made to the questions by those with dementia and those with depression. Definitive diagnosis cannot be made on the basis of these questions alone. Diagnosis requires a complete interview, discussed in more detail in Chapter 5, as well as a medical examination.

Where do you live?	Dementia: May confabulate, i.e., make up an answer, or be evasive. Depression: Will be able to give their most recent address with reasonable accuracy.
How is your health?	Dementia: May speak of a minor illness or deny any problems. Depression: May exhibit hysterical complaints, e.g., be very concerned about minor problems such as a cold.
How did you come here today?	Dementia: Will often refer to either an incorrect or inappropriate means of conveyance. Depression: Can give an accurate response.
Have you been nervous or anxious lately?	Dementia: Will usually deny any anxiety. Depression: Will usually indicate that it is part of their problem.

Once a complete evaluation has been performed and a diagnosis has been made, treatment may begin.

TREATMENT OF DEPRESSION AND DEMENTIA

While there are direct medical interventions for the cure of depression, there are none for dementia. In the dementias, however, there are interventions that can be made to control the individual's behavior. Regardless of the older adult's diagnosis, whether depression or dementia, interventions must follow a specified regimen. To begin with, treatment should be provided (1) in a warm, supportive atmosphere; (2) by a trained and caring individual; (3) on a regularly scheduled basis; and (4) when appropriate, with the involvement of other important individuals, such as family members.

Dementia: Reality Orientation

At present, physicians attempt to control the anxiety and agitation of dementia with medications. In addition, other health and social service providers attempt to encourage *reality orientation*, using methods based on the principles of behavior modification (Smith, Hanley-Germain, & Gips, 1971). This consists of a variety of techniques used to help an individual suffering from forgetfulness and confusion to slow the forgetting process and relearn important information. Several techniques are used to teach the information. These include repetition, sensory stimulation, and the use of cues.

At the most basic level, if people are to learn something new, they must pay attention to what they have to learn. With confused people, it is therefore necessary for the trainer constantly to redirect people back to the task at hand. Focusing attention can be done through the use of sensory stimulation. By playing music, spraying perfume, or gently touching people, their attention can be focused. Once their attention is focused on the learning task, repetition is used. It should be gentle and spaced over a few minutes (Baddeley, 1984). Finally, several external cues can be used. These can include notes on refrigerator doors, using color codes on doors, or using alarms as reminders for appointments (Kurlychek, 1983).

An important consideration for reality orientation is the question of *generalization*. In certain patients who attend reality-orientation programs in hospitals, clinics, or social service settings, it has been found that their memory skills are better at the reality-orientation program than when they return home. One reason might be that there is more social stimulation at the program than at home. Another is that the reality orientation learned at the program may not be directly applicable to what is needed at home (Brooks & Lincoln, 1984). The group leader should make every effort to see to it that the skills learned at the group can be useful elsewhere.

Reality orientation can and should be provided on a 24-hour basis. This is sometimes referred to as *milieu therapy* (Steer & Boyer, 1975). It is often conducted on a hospital or nursing home unit but can be performed successfully at home as well (Parker & Somers, 1983). The following are the procedures most often employed:

1. *Provide constant reminders* to the individual of their name, their caretakers' names, the time of day, the day of the week, and so forth. For example, say, "Hello Mr. Smith, I am Nurse Jones. Today is Monday. It is 11 o'clock in the morning, and we'll be having lunch at 12:30 in the dining room."

2. *Correct erroneous statements.* For example, say, "No Mr. Smith, this is not your home. It is the Midview Senior Center. Is there something about this place that reminds you of your home?"

3. *Announce activities* both before they take place and as they are about to happen. For example, say, "Mr. Smith, it is almost time for dinner. If you will take my hand I will escort you to the dining room so that we can have dinner."

4. *Minimize change.* Keep the confused person's belongings in the same place. Do not move furniture around.

5. *Get everyone involved.* It helps to keep a sense of pride.

Researchers hope one day to find a cure or technique to slow the deterioration of the brain in those suffering from dementia. Until such time, these techniques can help to keep the person oriented and involved.

Depression: Psychotherapy and Awareness Groups

Unlike dementia, if correctly diagnosed, depression can be treated very effectively. The more severe forms of depression can be treated with medications such as mood elevators and antidepressants. Most often, depression in the aged is treated by a combination of medication and psychotherapy. The aged, however, are often resistant to seeing a professional therapist. Traditionally, older adults have avoided psychotherapy (Gurlin, Veroff, & Field, 1960; U.S. General Accounting Office, 1982), seeking instead the aid of other family members, ministers, and physicians. This seems to be related to the fact that older adults themselves suffer from certain biases and fears. They may think that going to a therapist immediately labels them as crazy, they may see it as a sign of weakness.

It is important to note that sometimes when aged individuals go for psychotherapy they are brought in by others. The therapist is, therefore, seeing a person who may be very angry and resistant. Despite the resistance, several approaches to therapy with the aged have been used. A number of therapists recommend brief individual therapy or short-term counseling, to encourage the older person to become more involved with others. Social involvement reduces the loneliness and isolation that are part of depression (Croake & Glover, 1977).

Another method is the geriatric group approach. For example, a group might meet regularly for three hours each week. Part of the session could include a period devoted to listening to music chosen by a member of the group, followed by some breathing and movement exercises. The actual therapeutic session would not begin until a word game, a group form of free association, was initiated. According to the creators of this approach, their primary objectives are the "resocialization and reduction of isolation through increasing interpersonal verbal and nonverbal communication in the here and now" (Berger & Berger, 1971).

Another approach has been called the Geriatric Awareness Group Method. This begins with the advantage of being called an awareness group, rather than psychotherapy. This is helpful because, as we have said, older people have negative attitudes toward psychotherapy, and they may find it objectionable to divulge "secret" information to others they feel have not experienced things quite the way they have.

The awareness group brings together people who are of a similar age and tend to have similar experience, both in the past and present. Group work is also a natural way to counteract the passivity, low self-esteem, isolation, and resulting depression associated with aging. Even when you may not be able to force an individual to take an active part in a group, just coming to the group is a sign of activity and interest (Salamon, 1979).

Another important consideration is economics. An awareness group, while it may require supervision by a clinically trained therapist, does not necessarily require a group leader extensively trained in psychotherapeutic methods. The cost per person, therefore, is held down and the group is made appealing to prospective applicants. Since it is a group, the price for such a therapeutic service is lower than individual sessions.

In some other forms of group treatment, the therapist may take a passive role, encouraging socialization only as it becomes necessary. In the awareness group, the therapist/leader starts off by leading the discussions. The task of the leader in this awareness-group situation is to present the group with information regarding the relationships among loss, aging, and depression, just as a teacher might lead a class. The reason for this is that age and experience tend to give heightened insight. Just pointing out the problems sometimes will lead to rapid recognition and new strategies for coping. Another reason why the leader takes an active part in leading some of the discussions is that it gives the group members a chance to know each other better. They are given the opportunity to develop a sense of security and group cohesiveness.

The basic philosophy of the Geriatric Awareness Group is that as people age they lose some of life's positive reinforcers. Children, adolescents, and young adults can develop self-esteem around these societal reinforcers, which can then dwindle or change rapidly in later life, as people are faced with the traditional problems of the mature person, such as retirement, change of income level, widowhood, loneliness, and physical change. While these are radical changes, they can be compensated for from within the individual, via basic "life support" systems. These can be described best by example: If a person has devoted his entire life to work but now finds himself retired, he can either succumb to helpless feelings or rechannel the inner support system to a different kind of work. A typical recommendation that generally is effective in helping a person having difficulty in coping with retirement is to suggest that he volunteer to work in an organization that will appreciate his service. Even though the individual may not receive the secondary gain of being paid, he will be positively rewarded through appreciation of his efforts and accomplishments. The inner support system wants the individual to work and gain some reward for that work. The idea is to cope by channeling the system into another area of work that will be just as gratifying, and at a level the person can deal with.

The job of the Geriatric Awareness Group is to help the individual to tap her basic life support system through self-motivation and group dynamics. Each meeting, which lasts generally under two hours, deals with a specific loss, how it relates to the individuals in the group, and how they might best cope with it. Airing of the coping strategies of group members is encouraged. Discussion, the primary form of socialization, follows. The goal of the awareness group is to provide the depressed older adult with the ability to view things from a new perspective, with the support of others who encourage success.

LOVE AND GUILT: FAMILIES AND CRISIS INTERVENTION

We will begin this section with some case illustrations. A daughter who had lived with her mother until her late twenties, at which time she got married, brought her mother to live in her new house just a few days after the wedding. It took 20 more years of on-and-off therapy before the daughter, with her family's support, asked her mother, then in her late sixties, to move to a hotel for older adults. The daughter made all the arrangements and paid all the necessary fees. The mother went to the hotel somewhat begrudgingly and in a matter of a few short weeks began experiencing visual and auditory hallucinations. She expressed paranoid delusions to the staff of the hotel, became extremely depressed, and refused to leave her room. The hotel, unequipped to handle such cases, notified the daughter, who made arrangements for the mother to move back in with her. Because of her mother's condition, which did not exhibit itself after her return to her daughter's home, the daughter took an extended leave from her job. She felt that she had contributed to her mother's illness and wanted to make up for it.

At the other extreme is the child who deals with parental relationships by fleeing. A son who always had lived no more than a 10- to 15-minute walk from his parents' home decided to move 800 miles away two weeks following the death of his elderly father. He sold his business and home, telling his two sisters that the move was necessary for business reasons. He insisted that he was not running away from any responsibility; should his presence ever be needed, his sisters should not hesitate to call him. Inevitably, they did call him. Predictably, he completely shirked any responsibility, at times even refusing to return their phone calls. The sisters and elderly mother felt anger and annoyance at their brother and son, yet they exhibited it toward one another. The old woman became increasingly depressed until finally she refused to leave her house and answer her telephone, except when forced.

Another case is a woman in her early twenties who was living with her widowed mother. She was so afraid for her mother's health that she dressed her in the heaviest of sweaters, even on the hottest of days. She wouldn't turn on the air conditioner in the heat of summer for fear it might give her mother a cold. On days of inclement weather, the daughter would not let her elderly mother leave their apartment. The daughter would not let her nieces and nephews, the elder woman's grandchildren, kiss her mother for fear that she might pick up a germ. The mother and daughter constantly fought. The mother insisted that the daughter get married. The daughter refused to consider marriage, going so far as refusing evenings out with highly desirable men. The daughter stated that her primary responsibility was caring for her mother. The daughter's other siblings, while saying that they were concerned with their sister's dependence on their mother and apparent loss of individuality, were grateful that their mother was being attended to, in effect divorcing themselves from any and all responsibility. They felt comfortable visiting two or three times a month to check up on their mother's progress. The mother, meanwhile, was hardly ever ill. The most serious illness she had experienced in the previous five years was a mild bout of influenza.

Another problem that inevitably arises is who will make the decision regarding nursing home placement for an elderly parent. Children, mature in all their other dealings, show up in an agitated state, hoping—praying in fact—that the health care professional will remove the burden of decision from their shoulders. It is not uncommon for children to trick elderly parents into nursing home placement. One hears of cases of children dropping their parents off at nursing homes without any warning.

The preceding cases are typical samples of the kind of difficulties a person working in the field of gerontology is asked to deal with on a regular basis. Most of the presenting problems of the elderly are not individual problems but involve a larger social sphere. Sometimes even neighbors become involved. The job, then, for the health and social workers providing services to the elderly is not simply to diagnose the problem of an elder family member but to mediate among family members, to provide an environment in which solutions can be achieved to the best interests of all. (Some of these issues will be discussed further in Chapter 5.)

It is not the worker's task to make decisions for the family, but it is the professional's task to deal with them in an effective manner. Toward this end there are a few major principles that should be kept in mind:

1. Communication between parents and children, and between children and their siblings, should be reality bound, not based on traditions or historical pecking orders, or prompted by manipulation and a sense of guilt.
2. The thoughts of the parents always should be taken into consideration. It is not uncommon for the children to have a family meeting to decide on what is to be done about the elderly parent, without even consulting the parent. This behavior should be confronted and discouraged.
3. All options should be discussed. For example, is the parent really a nursing home candidate, or is it realistic to arrange for home care?

Children often decide for their parents that they want to have their parents living in a different neighborhood. Perhaps they feel the neighborhood is just not safe enough. The children get together and find an apartment and come to the parents to announce the joyous news. Much to their dismay, their parents think that they have done them a terrible misdeed, and in fact the parents have been struck a serious blow to their self-esteem. The result usually is that both the parents and children are hurt.

In dealing with a situation of this nature, one looks for the options. Are there programs in the neighborhood in which the parents live that provide services for them that they are not aware of? Is there a buddy system that might be arranged, perhaps through the local police precinct or social service agency, to provide a more watchful eye and greater degree of security for the patients? These are just two of the many possible options. It is the task of the gerontologist to explore these options.

As some of the preceding examples indicate, the problems go deeper than just dealing with the elderly family member. One of the major factors in depression among the aged is social. The family is still one of the primary social spheres. Toward this end, it is often the task of the professional to deal with unfinished development on the part of the adult children. Adult children often have ambivalent, immature, or even hostile ties with their parents. A child who deals in guilt with a parent cannot be in a position to truly provide the help an older parent may need.

The best method of dealing with the family problem must be found. A group method or family therapy may be beneficial. It would be a wise choice of action if, once the immediate problem has been addressed, the adult children are taught to understand what caused the problem initially, how it was dealt with, and why the new course of action was decided upon. While the emphasis in this work is on the aged family member, it is important to deal with the social environment too, especially children and other close relatives.

SUMMARY

This chapter has reviewed the most common forms of mental health problems in the aged, including a review of the psychological and sociological components of personality and the roles most frequently observed in the aged. In addition, the social, environmental, and biological stresses of aging were examined, with an eye toward their impact on well-being in the aged. Recognizing when an older adult is suffering from a mental disorder is an important skill for health and social workers to acquire. Being able to distinguish between types of illness is an even more significant skill. It is necessary to recognize symptoms, understand their causes, and prepare care interventions. This chapter introduced the reader to these tasks and roles. Chapter 5 will offer further techniques. But before it is possible to intervene with specific individuals, programs usually need to be in place, and the first step in establishing such programs is an assessment of what important needs may be going unmet within the community. The following chapter explores the assessment process.

4

How to Assess Community Needs

Needs assessment is an attempt to explain or understand the demands a specific segment of society places on a service provider. A segment of society can be defined geographically, ethnically, or by age. There are three basic steps in needs assessment: (1) identifying the problems, (2) prioritizing the problems, and (3) identifying relevant services and where they are provided. Since we have already discussed types of services and where they are provided in Chapters 1 and 2, this chapter will focus on techniques for identifying and prioritizing need.

Nationwide, the more than 600 state and area agencies on aging are required by law to know the needs of the elderly residing in their communities (U.S. Federal Register, 1973). It is recognized, however, that the agencies have yet to fulfill this mandate (U.S. Federal Register, 1979). While methods of assessment are generally known, individuals who understand their importance are wanting. This is just one reason why those working with the elderly must be familiar with needs assessment methodologies. Another reason is that assessment and evaluation (as discussed in Chapter 8) use similar tools. Assessing whether a program is operating according to the specifications and is meeting a need is an important job for gerontologists.

SURVEYING A COMMUNITY

There are a number of techniques that may be used to assess the needs of a community, but first the need that is going to be examined must be clearly defined. What we mean by this is best explained by example. If we wanted to know the number of homebound elderly who reside in an area, would we be referring to those individuals who are bedridden in their own homes or to those who can walk short distances with the assistance of a prosthetic device such as a walker? Are we interested because we want to know how many need the services of a visiting nurse or how many need help with cleaning their homes or apartments once a week? Clearly, there is a broad range of possibilities. It is also conceivable that we want information on all of these issues, but how do we go about finding out the answers? The first step must be to delineate clearly what we wish to know.

Once the issue to be examined has been clearly specified and understood, there are a number of techniques we can use. In our case, let us assume that we want to know how many homebound elderly there are in the community so that we can plan for a home-delivered meal program. In this type of situation, our definition of homebound may be somewhat relaxed. The homebound individual need not be entirely restricted to bed but would be considered homebound if incapacitated to the point of being unable to prepare one major, nutritious meal a day. An additional requirement we may have is that no one is available to assist the homebound individual with the preparation of such a meal. Before examining how to assess this particular need, let us take a look at the techniques that are available to the practitioner.

Techniques

Needs assessment techniques can be divided into a number of different categories. Some investigators suggest that there are as many as seven distinct techniques for needs assessment (Larcau & Heumann, 1982). Others (Warheite, Bell, & Schwab, 1974) suggest that there are only four. In fact, the distinction is simply semantic, for a number of techniques can be subsumed under one methodological approach.

The four general techniques for needs assessment we will use are (1) gathering opinions, (2) collecting service statistics, (3) appraising social indicators, and (4) making surveys.

Gathering Opinions and Judgments. This process includes a number of techniques for seeking out information from individuals familiar with the topic under study. One method is known as the *key informant* or knowledgeable person approach. The individuals selected to provide information on the needs of the group are assumed to have firsthand knowledge of the services available within the community. They are also known to have familiarity with the group under scrutiny. Often, in older-adult needs assessments, these individuals are politicians or administrators of both public and private institutions serving the elderly population. Another good source of key informants is the local government department for aging services. In order to record accurately the information that key individuals offer, the use of a structured interview is recommended. Such an interview has predetermined goals and questions. Using key informants is advantageous for two reasons. First, it is relatively inexpensive to perform, and second, by involving key community leaders, it offers a good public relations function. It does, however, have one major drawback: Despite the fact that a good many community leaders are surveyed, it is only their biases, or the positions of the organizations that they represent, that are recorded. Their position may not represent adequately the full range of needs of the older individuals of the community.

Another method that is used to gather opinions regarding the needs of the elderly is the *public forum*. In this approach, a large group of community residents is invited to attend a forum to discuss the needs of the community. In the sense that it provides a forum for individual views, it is similar to the key informant technique. It is a somewhat stronger approach in that a wider range of community dwellers is invited to present information to the researchers. To the degree that forum participants are representatives of the community, this technique can be effective. One important note is that when this type of needs assessment is undertaken, it is important to advertise the meeting widely and see to it that the participation is reflective of the community. It is necessary to arrange transportation to the forum, for the homebound; otherwise, it is doubtful whether their opinions would be adequately represented.

A further method is the *group process*. In this approach, a number of individuals get together to brainstorm and exchange ideas. One formal method of group process is the *nominal groups approach*. In this technique, members of the group are asked to list all the possible responses to an open-ended question. An example might be, "How can the nutritional needs of the homebound elderly of Anaconda County be met?" The group participants are then asked to list all the nonrepetitive responses and prioritize them. This approach allows for the summing of responses resulting in a priority compilation of needs. The disadvantages of this approach are similar to those listed for the other methods of gathering opinions and judgments; namely, are the members of the group who are taking part in the assessment representative of the individuals whose needs are being addressed?

One further disadvantage of all opinion-gathering techniques that must be guarded against is the raising of expectations that a group process or public forum will immediately result in a program to meet the needs that are documented. It is the task of the surveyor to spell out clearly the goals of the assessment. This type of evaluation is not results oriented; rather, it is decision oriented. Goals should be limited to the acquisition of relevant data and the compilation of a final report. Whether or not a program designed to respond to the findings results from the assessment is an issue the surveyor cannot address.

Collecting Service Statistics. There are two sources of service statistics. The first is known as *rates under treatment*, or service user records. The second is called *service request records. Rates under treatment* is an enumeration of those individuals who have utilized services in a community. This information comes from the case records of service providers. The assumption of this approach is that, if individuals request more service than can be provided, then a *prima facie* case exists for providing that service. If, however, services are underutilized, then the program size can be reduced.

While this method is inexpensive and widely used, it has a number of drawbacks. First, the surveyors must not violate the confidentiality of the service recipient. When information is given to a service provider, it is given with the assumption that no one else will see that individual's records. Steps to insure confidentiality, such as removing any identifying information, must be taken. A second drawback is that this technique does not provide a measure of unmet needs. It identifies only the number of individuals receiving the service, not those who are not. Further, it cannot account for any possible duplication of service where, as often occurs, one individual receives the same type of assistance from more than one provider.

The *service request record* method of collecting service statistics attempts to control for the shortcomings of the *rates under treatment* approach. By examining the requests for assistance, the surveyor can determine whether or not the need is great. This method too, is relatively inexpensive but has additional drawbacks. Few organizations keep records of the number of individuals who seek a service they do not provide. Furthermore, it is difficult to know if the number of calls requesting a service reflect a few callers who try repeatedly to receive assistance, or if many different individuals are calling. An additional drawback is that, here too, this method cannot measure unmet need. If a program were introduced and properly advertised, it is conceivable that many more individuals would require the service and take steps to request it. But, until it is in place, these individuals must find other ways of responding to their needs.

Social Indicators Technique. Sometimes referred to as the social indicator method, this is based on the use of available records, usually census data. Vast amounts of data exist on the elderly, and they can provide a great deal of information as to where older adults live, what services they use, and even future need projections of the elderly. Here, too, this technique is a relatively inexpensive one. The drawback here is the indirectness of the measurement. This is a major shortcoming in that it may result in inaccurate conclusions. Furthermore, it is not uncommon to assume mistakenly that there is a causal relationship between the characteristics of the individuals from whom data were obtained and their needs. Just because someone is old does not necessarily mean that they need assistance. Another factor is that, by the time census data become available, they are usually out of date. There is no reason to assume that a level of need reported in the past will pertain to the present or, especially, to the future.

Surveys. Often used as means of assessing the needs of the community, *respondent surveys* elicit information from the individuals with the most information—those for whom programs are being planned. There are generally three methods used: (1) the face-to-face approach, (2) the telephone survey, and (3) the mail survey.

The face-to-face approach is primarily an interview, usually involving a structured questionnaire. When working with the elderly, it is important to remember that the individual must be placed at ease (see Chapter 5), so interviewing is best done at a location where the respondent is comfortable. Confidentiality must be assured, especially when asking questions regarding sensitive matters. The discussion should be clear and its purpose well spelled out. It is important to develop a sense of how long the interview period should run. For some older individuals a face-to-face interview may be the only human contact they have had in days. They may therefore seek to prolong it. In other cases, elderly individuals may quickly tire of the questions. Both instances require a warm interview style, with attention to the questions to be addressed and the clients' needs.

While it used to be assumed that the face-to-face approach was the best method of collecting valid, accurate data, there is accumulating evidence that indicates that both the telephone and the mail survey methods are just as effective in obtaining data (LaCherie et al., 1981; Leinbach, 1982). In these approaches, a brief questionnaire is designed and tested for reliability to see if it gathers information in a consistent manner. It is then mailed to a representative sample of the elderly residing in an area, or answers are solicited via telephone. Two possible disadvantages occur when using either the mail or telephone. Once again, the issue of representativeness arises. Are those older individuals who receive the questionnaire truly representative of the members of the older-adult community being surveyed? For instance, do all older adults in the community have telephones? Do they read their own mail or have to wait for someone to assist them with it? While methods of sampling for representativeness are beyond the scope of this book, suffice it to say that when a random selection procedure is used the question of representativeness is reduced (see Sudman, 1976).

An additional concern that often arises regarding non face-to-face interviews is whether or not self-report can be considered completely accurate. This is particularly a problem for mail interviews, where even voice contact with the respondent is lacking. In addition to finding accumulating evidence that self-report is valid in a variety of situations (Hickey, 1980; Linn & Linn, 1980), interviewers' biases are bypassed when using this approach, and it may therefore be used without much fear of inaccuracy.

First Steps

Before undertaking any needs assessment of older adults, it is important to keep in mind the special problems posed by older adult communities. Among these are the larger percentage of women at increasing ages. It is important to specify age groups and gender representation in the assessment. Where the elderly reside is an additional issue of vital importance. Rural elderly, in general, are older and more isolated, have been living in the same place longer, have more serious transportation problems, and have lower incomes than city-dwelling elders (Auerbach, 1972). Specifying the type of community and the general services available is important. The items to be specified include transportation and even the existence of public sewer systems. It also may be important to look at the rates of illness of the group being examined, to determine whether these are factors in defining and responding to need. An additional aspect of importance is the ethnic breakdown of the elderly community being studied. While the minority elderly constitute only 10 percent of the U.S. population over age 65, they have an overall quality of life that is, on the average, well below nonminority elderly. When the specific issues of the survey are clearly stated and prioritized, we can then start to examine the problem.

If we use as an example the task of assessing the need of the homebound elderly so as to plan for their nutritional requirements, before we decide on which technique to use, we should take a closer look at the community. Suppose we find that the community is a rural one. Most of the homes are very old and are set back from the main road and there is no public transportation available. We also find the elderly community dwellers to be generally nonwhite and quite poor.

There are some additional features for us to consider in our survey. Are there service providers in the community? In fact, we find that there is a senior citizens center centrally located and only about a 25-minute car ride from the furthest older adult. Are these individuals truly homebound? We would want to look at the types of chronic illnesses in this particular older-adult community and determine whether they truly restrict residents' mobility. In this instance the community is a small one, so we opt for direct, face-to-face interviews and decide to look at an additional aspect—the support systems available to the older adults of this community.

DEVELOPING AND IMPLEMENTING PROGRAMS

Knowing what type of program should be developed, where to implement it, and how best to keep it going requires planning on a variety of levels. Some aspects of planning have been discussed already. These include translating the information obtained from the needs assessment stage into useful programming ideas. Morris and Binstock (1966) suggest that there are five stages in program planning. The first three stages have been reviewed in the needs assessment section: (1) identification of the problem, (2) undertaking a study to analyze the problem, and (3) involvement of the vested interests, as might be done in a community forum or face-to-face approach. The final two stages are (4) the development of a plan of action and (5) implementing the planned program.

All planning schemes must consider the long-term impact or goals of the program and also the short-term objectives. Short-term objectives help us to establish priorities along the way toward achieving the long-term goals. Short-term objectives generally are measurable in the sense that one can state concretely whether or not these objectives have been achieved. Long-term goals, however, may not be as readily measured. In our case example, the long-term goal of our project might very well be to increase the rates of socialization and thereby lower the levels of loneliness of the homebound, rural elderly in our study. One short-term objective toward reaching that goal might be to inform all the residents of the availability of the senior citizen program. In this case, the objective can be readily measured. If every older adult has been notified, we have succeeded in our short-term objective. It will take quite a lot more to determine whether the long-term goal has been achieved.

One more issue crucial to the development of programming for the elderly is how the project will be funded. Planning for this stage is of major importance. Will the program be funded by government monies, church funds, or by membership fees? Without first evaluating the availability and adequacy of funding, one may not reasonably undertake to implement a program.

OUTREACH

Placing a telephone call to each of the rural elderly residents in our survey community is one form of outreach. Outreach is, by definition, the act or process of reaching out to individuals or groups to inform them about, make them aware of, and encourage them to become interested in a program or project. There is more, however. It includes locating the target group in order to inform them properly of the program. If all of the residents of our example rural community owned telephones, then outreach via telephone might be a viable option. In large urban areas, though, not only is it difficult to call all the targeted individuals, but it may be impossible to know just how many of the group actually live in the area. This is perhaps one of the reasons why, as valuable programs for the elderly have been developed, only a small proportion of the estimated eligible members of the target groups have taken part in these services.

Another possible reason for the small proportion of older adults involved in services designed for their benefit is that many of the current population of elderly tend to be fiercely independent and consider it degrading to seek assistance from human service providers, except perhaps in time of dire need. Outreach that informs people before a need becomes critical and is beyond assistance is important. It is also clear that outreach must include more than just simple advertising of program availability.

Some straightforward methods of outreach include distributing flyers and pamphlets about a program to community residents. This is usually accompanied by letters of introduction to other service professionals in the area, alerting them to the program. If other professionals become aware of the program, they can act as referral sources. Individuals who work for local hospitals, public health services, community action programs, and similar projects are good contacts in the outreach process.

One major drawback to contacting human service providers is that they, too, service only a limited number of elderly. To increase the possibility of contacting more older adults, church groups should be included in the outreach effort, but here, too, only a limited number of individuals will be reached. Direct service providers may be an even better source for disseminating information regarding a new program. Police officers, mail carriers, grocers, druggists, and even physicians often have a great deal of contact with the isolated elderly (Salamon & Nichol, 1982). Also, not to be discounted are barber shops, beauticians, work supervisors, and even bartenders, all of whom often have more direct input with those in need than social service professionals (Cowens, 1982).

Perhaps the most effective way to reach the difficult-to-find elderly is through what is sometimes referred to as the snowball technique. This involves using informal support networks to notify those who can be reached. Those contacted would be asked to tell their friends, neighbors, and relatives about the program or service, thus geometrically expanding the outreach effort.

Both the use of the public media—newspapers, radio, and television—and door-to-door canvassing as techniques of outreach are widely recommended; however, these approaches are limited in their usefulness. Because many older adults do not always have access to television or even radio, and because many find it difficult to read the small print in newspapers, they tend not to be cognizant of outreach advertising. Door-to-door canvassing is not a cost-effective method of outreach because it requires a great deal of time and effort. Even when housing information is combined with census-tract data in locating the elderly, there is no guarantee that you can gain the attention of the elderly you wish to reach. A flyer slipped under a door or placed in a mailbox may go unnoticed at best. In urban areas, very few elderly will allow strangers into their homes to explain a new program to them and perform outreach. Using senior volunteers is another possible outreach approach. Older-adult volunteers are trained to go out into the community and assist in locating peers who could benefit from the program, at which time they explain the program to them. This has proven to be one successful approach (Terris, 1977).

VESTED INTERESTS

One major aspect of the program-development process is the involvement of vested interests in the planning stage. We have noted previously that this process is part of community forums. While this is one possible method for encouraging involvement of vested interests, it is by no means the only one, nor should it be considered the most beneficial. Community input is of course quite valuable in the assessment of needs, but for the planning and development of new programs that are designed to respond to the needs found in the assessment stage, the input of vested interests is vital.

In our case example of the rural, homebound elderly, involving vested community interests could be the deciding factor determining whether or not our goals might ever be reached. Let us assume from our example that we can safely state that we have been successful in achieving our first short-term objective, which was to telephone all the elderly residents of the community. We also are confident that we have explained clearly to them the relative proximity of the local senior citizens center and of the value of the programming offered there. Now that we have succeeded in providing the community residents with the appropriate information and can hope that we have aroused their interest, how can we assist them in getting to the senior center? If we involve the vested interests of the community and are somewhat creative in our approach, we may be successful.

Suppose we discover that the local church owns a school bus that is used to transport the same homebound older adults to Sunday morning services. It would be wise, then, for a variety of reasons, to involve the church in the planning and program development process. We might find that the church bus is not used on Mondays, Wednesdays, and Fridays, and the church leadership, mindful of the importance of senior center involvement for the elderly residents of the community, is willing to offer the bus to transport the residents to the center. The church however, cannot afford to pay for the services of a bus driver. A number of suggestions may be offered, including asking a school bus driver to assist following completion of rounds with school children. Other possibilities include involving local merchants, asking for donations from the rural residents themselves, or seeking governmental assistance.

In this case example there proves to be an overriding general interest on the part of the community to provide services to older adults. Also, advance planning was done. This, however, is not always the case. In the two examples that follow, issues of territoriality and problems with overlapping programs work to hinder the service provider from performing their task.

One example involves a program funded through government grants. The typical method of evaluating the effectiveness of the project is through the number of service units, which means that the major thrust often is more on the number of people serviced than on the actual client who receives the service. This example is of a suburban community with a very high percentage of elderly residents. Within this community, four government-funded senior centers exist to service the needs of the elderly community residents. All have similar programs, and all of the centers have the same names on their membership rosters; that is, most of the community elderly who belong to senior centers belong not to just one but all four. Poor community planning may have been the cause in this situation, though it is clear that a high proportion of the older adults who could use the services of the centers simply do not. Outreach has not been extensively performed in this neighborhood. In addition to in-house programs for recreation, socialization, and nutrition, all four centers have meals-on-wheels programs, which are designed to provide the truly homebound of the community with one hot, nutritious meal per day. All are government funded.

At some sites, the funding allows for the preparation and delivery of a relatively few daily meals, while at the other sites more than a few meals are prepared. The total government funding for meals on wheels in the community is 100 meals per day. It was found that many of the elderly, through no fault of their own, were on the meals-on-wheels list at more than one center. In fact, while 100 meals were prepared, only 70 people were receiving them. Some individuals obviously received more than the one meal allotted to them. It took a good number of years for this fact to become known to the service providers, despite the fact that some of the homebound seniors questioned why they received more than one meal. Even then, it took a while before the overlap was acknowledged as a problem.

To overcome the problem, it took the resourcefulness of the service providers and their ability to join together to find ways of coping with the issue. In this instance, it was found that even more of the elderly of the community could be serviced if the four centers joined together. The result was that resources were pooled. The center with the largest food-preparation capacity prepared all the meals. The center with the largest professional staff was charged with outreach, intake, and follow-up, to determine if those who applied for the program were truly needy. Once a person was approved for service, the staff of this center were charged with seeing to it that meals were delivered on time. The two remaining centers provided the transportation services that brought the meals from the preparation site to the individual's home.

This is an example of a relatively straightforward resolution to a problem. In other cases, resolutions to the problem of territoriality are not as easy to arrive at.

Senior gathering places, in particular senior centers, are rapidly becoming focal points for the delivery of a variety of services to the elderly (Jacobs, 1980). One of these services is related to the health needs of the participants. In some centers, programs run jointly by the local older-adult agency and a hospital provide regular medical screenings. These health fairs act as an early warning method and are designed to forestall severe health problems by recognizing in early stages. In a number of instances similar programs have met with a great deal of opposition from local medical professionals (Kos, 1976; Salamon, Charytan, McQuade & Friedman, 1982), as they often have been seen as being a threat to the medical community. The local health providers are unsure of the merits of the program and are worried about the effects it may have on their patients. In addition, they might find it threatening in the sense that they may lose their patients to a different health service program, and they may see it as a negative indicator of their ability. They reason that the present medical services are sufficient, so why bring in others?

To overcome this antagonism, extensive public education must be undertaken by the new program's staff and the service providers already in place. The educational component should begin even before the new program has started. Describing what was found during the needs-assessment stage, explaining the analysis of the need, and then involving these providers in the actual program planning could help alleviate some of the difficulty. While we are hopeful that using this approach would help to overcome some of the territoriality problems, it would be naïve to assume that it will always be successful. In fact, each program has its own needs, which result from its operating guidelines, financial situation, and the particular needs of those being serviced. Even when agreement for cooperation has been reached, there is no guarantee that it will continue. Regular follow-up meetings in which the program's development is discussed should be mandated. Yet this too does not assure the ongoing cooperation needed for success. Perhaps the only real signal of program success is when the long-term goals of a project show signs of being reached. This may take a long time. If, however, the assessment and the program planning have been carried out properly, and if the outreach program has been well targeted, then those who need the service should begin to receive it, and that should be one of the best measures of success.

FUNCTIONS OF THE INFORMATION-AND-REFERRAL PROCESS

Information-and-referral programs began in the late ninteenth century in the United States and England. Social and charitable service providers, as a way to avoid duplication of their efforts and to improve the efficiency of the client screening process, centralized their information on available services and thereby streamlined the referral process. In the mid twentieth century, Community Chests sought a way of increasing the visibility of the programs they helped to fund. The technique they used included the development of formal information-and-referral units (McCaslin, 1981). Individuals with a human need question could call the information number, where a telephone counselor would refer the person to the appropriate service provider.

All social service programs have an information-and-referral component. Once a program has begun to operate and has notified potential clients of its existence via successful outreach, interested clients or consumers of the service have to be brought into the system. This intake process may be initiated by either the service provider or the client, but it always begins with the information-and-referral step. A potential client, having heard of the program, may call or write for more information. This request for information may go directly to the service provider or to a referral agency; in any case, it is at this step that the process has begun.

McCaslin (1981), in a survey of the literature, found that there are primarily four functions included in the information-and-referral process: (1) providing information, (2) steering, (3) giving advice, and (4) making a referral. To these we will add (5) recording, (6) follow-up, (7) advocacy, and (8) the ombudsman role.

Providing Information

Information giving can be seen as the first extension of the outreach process. Providing information to interested parties can be done simply by dispensing telephone numbers, or it may be more actively performed by investing a good deal of effort in searching out the precise resources that provide for a client's specific needs.

When individuals respond to information-and-referral services, particularly the elderly who find it difficult to admit to a need for aid, they should not simply be turned away if the program they contacted does not provide for their specific needs. Older-adult programs should develop and maintain comprehensive community resource files. To do this, the worker needs to survey the programs available in a community. Some of this information may be available already from the needs-assessment phase. In some communities, political organizations have listings of various service providers that can be used for referrals. The resource file also should include information on informal service providers. In our example of the rural, homebound elderly, we might have found that some community teenagers had taken to shopping for the older residents, providing this service after school, for a small fee. This service, though not government sponsored, is a valuable resource.

Steering

Resource files must be well organized so that everyone using the file has the pertinent information at their fingertips. Index cards cross-referenced by name and services provided are recommended. When a caller requests information, the information-and-referral service can then direct or steer the client to the program by simply informing the caller of a specific programs existence.

Giving Advice

A third function of the information-and-referral process is giving advice. The worker indicates to the client, in an objective manner, which might be the better course of action to take in responding to the client's needs. Salamon and Grodin (1982) have suggested that, due to the increasing complexity of society and its technologies, the gerontology service professional must help the potential client to make rapid yet accurate decisions. By doing so, entry into the system is quickly initiated.

Making a Referral

The referral function takes place when the information-and-referral worker actually contacts the service-providing agency to schedule a contact or meeting with the client. In order to do this, the contact usually must contain a form of assessment in which the client's needs are accurately determined. A number of studies indicate that the more active the service professional is in making the referral, the more likely it is that the client will make contact with the agency referred to. Individuals who are actively referred are more likely to continue contact, as opposed to those clients who are simply steered and told of a service program's existence (Kogan, 1957; Parnicky, Anderson, Nakoa, & Thomas, 1961).

Gaitz, McCaslin, and Calvert (1977) have suggested that the information-and-referral process includes more than just providing details of a service program to an interested caller. As we have seen, the request for service is not necessarily the type of service actually needed. Because of this, the counselor must ascertain whether or not the stated need is the real one. If not, the information-and-referral counselor should evaluate the client further before recommending service.

There also may exist a treatment component in the form of providing assurances or counseling to the caller. This is particularly the case in hotline information-and-referral programs. Callers may be agitated or fearful and may require the immediate skills of a counseling professional. Counseling clients via telephone may be an asset when working with the elderly, becausc, while face-to-face contact may be lacking, individual personal contact is not, and telephone counseling is one means of overcoming the transportation problem so often faced by older adults.

Recording

Regardless of how far the information-and-referral process goes in its efforts, all requests for information should be recorded accurately, including

1. When the contact was made or the call received
2. Who made the contact, including whether it was an older adult, a neighbor, or a family member
3. The type of service requested
4. Whether or not the service requested seemed appropriate to meeting the stated need
5. What, if any, service or referral could be provided

This information is invaluable when performing a needs assessment. It also might be indicative of poor outreach. When few requests for assistance come in, it may be assumed that those who need the service have not been informed of its existence. It also might indicate that the outreach effort was misdirected, as when it is found that several requests for service come in that reflect a misunderstanding of the program. By recording information on requests for service, greater insight into community structure may be gained, including who the underserved are, where they reside, and what their needs are. Also, duplication of services or gaps in service provision may be discovered.

Follow-up

An important component of any information-and-referral program is follow-up. Sometimes all of the cases are followed up by either calling the agency to whom the client was referred or calling the client to ascertain if contact for service was made. In some programs, a few randomly selected cases are chosen for follow-up and are used as a representative sample of all the cases. In any event, the information obtained from follow-up is valuable and adds to the data obtained at the initial contact.

Advocacy

When the information-and-referral worker actively assists clients in obtaining their rights and services, particularly when other service agencies do not readily provide the service, the worker acts as an advocate. An advocate is someone who pleads the case of another. Advocacy for elderly clients occurs in a variety of situations, not simply through the information-and-referral process. As we have seen, older adults tend not to initiate contact or even be aware of service providers and the programs they offer. They are even less likely to challenge service providers or agencies that do not provide them with the service they require. There are times when this procedure takes on the nature of a "catch-22" situation. Some service programs require that older adults fill out forms or otherwise provide an agency with extensive amounts of information before they can be evaluated for the service. At the same time, however, the older adult does not know where to obtain the information requested or does not know or understand how to fill out the necessary forms. The agency may not offer assistance in this initial process. The role of an advocate in this setting would be to help the older adult with consolidating the necessary data or to attempt to have the contact agency assist the older adult with the procedure. Whenever the rights of independence, well-being, care, and protection of older adults are violated, advocacy is required. There are several basic strategies that may be applied.

Gaining Broad Support. The most general strategy and perhaps the most useful in the long run is to gain a broad base of support. On the level of large groups, the advocacy role may include lobbying politicians to support policies that are more sympathetic to the needs of the elderly. On the individual case level, broad-based support can be obtained by discussing the problem at case conferences or service-provider councils at which various agencies are represented.

Becoming Familiar with the System. The advocate must be knowledgeable about the system or organization that will be challenged. For example, if a landlord is evicting elderly tenants in order to be able to charge higher rents, it is the role of the advocate to understand housing laws and tenants' rights.

Involving Professionals. It is also important to involve professionals in areas of their expertise. In some cases, this might include attorneys and legislators. One approach is to find out if other professionals are already involved as advocates, and, if they are, to work with them in a unified manner.

Confronting. Confrontation between an advocate and an organization occurs regularly. To overcome the anger and work toward an acceptable solution requires diplomacy and the ability not to get discouraged.

Protecting the Client. Perhaps the most important aspect of advocacy is protecting the most vulnerable individual in the process—the older client—from any more violations or insults. This might require the advocate to protect the name of the individual represented until all necessary assurances for confidentiality are made.

Maintaining Client Independence. Advocates can go too far. It is wise for advocates to evaluate the ability of their clients to take care of their own needs. Advocates should never allow clients to become so dependent on professional assistance that they cannot take part in the proceedings on their own behalf.

Performing the Ombudsman Role. There are, however, individuals who cannot fend for themselves, for example, seriously ill people in nursing homes. There have been scores of reports of patient abuse and poor care in long-term care facilities (U.S. Senate, 1974–

1976). One means of providing advocacy that has evolved recently is the ombudsman program. There are three roles an ombudsman may take (Monk & Kaye, 1982):

1. Impartial mediator, arbitrating between the patient and the staff or administration of the facility
2. Active disputant, taking the client's side when necessary to achieve change
3. Giver of emotional support, propping up the weaker party so that she or he does not suffer more undue discomfort

All three roles are required on various occasions, with the ultimate goal being the improvement of the client's quality of life.

SUMMARY

This chapter was a review of the methods and techniques used to identify and prioritize needs of the community-dwelling elderly. In addition some basic sampling techniques were examined. Some ways of developing formal support programs and having them operate successfully were presented with special emphasis placed on planning and outreach. The goal of all these efforts is to improve well-being and quality of life for older adults. Many of these programs, however, in turn depend on the worker's ability to interview individual older adults. Whether the goal is to assess unmet needs or to evaluate currently provided services, workers need to know what to ask and how to ask it. The next chapter examines how to conduct a successful interview.

5

How to Interview Older Adults

The idea for this chapter grew out of a desire to provide a concrete, structured approach for interviewing the elderly. Many texts contain references to general techniques of interviewing (Brink, 1979; Kane & Kane, 1981; Schlossberg & Entine, 1978; Storandt, 1983). Few, however, provide formal details and case studies. This chapter consists of a conceptual overview, some detailed techniques, and specific examples of the first meeting and subsequent information-gathering sessions between an interviewer and an older adult client.

All too often, we have the impression that interviews must be conducted in a rather brief period of time. We therefore tend to sacrifice the development of rapport for the sake of accuracy. An unfortunate consequence is that we hurry the process, display our anxiety with the rushing clock, and make the client feel ill at ease. The result is incomplete or inaccurate information in our records. Because treatment plans are often developed from this information, it is not rare for us to find that we are having difficulty in accurately responding to the client's real needs. While time pressure is a real phenomenon, there are techniques that the interviewer may use to his/her advantage. This chapter will explain ways of starting an interview, listening to what is being said, and understanding the underlying implications. It also lists a number of structured and semistructured approaches to interviewing. While no one approach is described, general techniques, some statements, and responses often heard, and some accepted interventions are explored in a way that will help both the novice and more experienced interviewer to understand better the process of interviewing older adults.

RAPPORT: PUTTING THE CLIENT AT EASE

When assessments are performed for the very first time with an older-adult client, the client is usually fearful of the process. This is true even when the older adult has been well prepared for the interview by his or her family. There is often a fear on the client's part that "something will be wrong" or "they will put me away."

The result of an older-adult client's fear of the interview is often a defensiveness that may be expressed by acting out, either through anger and hostility or through indifference. Defensiveness is exhibited by reactions such as "It's none of your business" or "I know but won't tell you." Sometimes defensiveness is exhibited by an almost complete malleability. An example of this is the client who comes to the interview well prepared with shopping bags of important papers and will not respond to a question without first asking the interviewer to check these papers.

None of these negative reactions are conducive to an information gathering session. The interviewer, therefore, must move quickly to put the client at ease, as misleading behaviors resulting from trepidation on the part of the client can lead to inaccurate diagnoses. The acting-out individual may be seen as a "dangerous" or argumentative client, while the passively hostile individual may be thought to have a mental impairment, an inability to remember, or signs of perseveration, a neurotic characteristic. It is the interviewer's responsibility to go beyond the defensiveness resulting from a healthy fear to the real, underlying issue. It is also important to be able to distinguish between normal reactions and psychopathological trepidation.

There are a number of ways to put an older-adult client at ease (Weiner, Brok, & Snadowsky, 1978). These include the use of language, physical contact, and posturing or body language. It is also important to show respect, understanding for the client's preferences and capacities.

Language

Many interviewers refer to older-adult clients by their first names. There has been much talk about the importance and appropriateness of this technique. Many argue that calling someone by their first name creates an immediate feeling of camaraderie. Not only is this an inaccurate assumption, but it also can be deleterious in its effect (Salamon, 1979). A young physician may feel secure enough in her position to call a new patient, old enough to be her grandmother, by her first name. The patient will likely resent the doctor for taking that liberty with her prestige. She may correctly feel that by virtue of her age alone she deserves the respect of being called by her full name.

Calling individuals by their title, such as Mr., Ms., or Dr., suggests very clearly that respect is being accorded to the client. Interviewers should not make light of this and should call an individual by her first name only if the client suggests that it is acceptable.

Physical Contact

Many students of psychotherapy question whether or not physical contact with a client is appropriate. The fear of *transference*, wherein an unrealistic relationship develops between the client and therapist, is the reason for the frowning upon of contact. Transference, however, can have a beneficial component as well. It is important for a client to feel that a special relationship does exist with the therapist or interviewer. If this does not take place, the client will not feel sufficiently at ease to divulge to a stranger what may be considered very private information. Transference in working with older adults usually takes the form of seeing a similarity between the interviewer and a relative of the client. Examples include "You remind me of my grandson" or "I have a beautiful granddaughter, well educated. Are you married? Maybe you have a single brother?" As this form of transference is the most common, some physical contact in the form of a handshake or placing a comforting hand on the clients' shoulder can be acceptable. If the client displays sexual transference of a pathological nature, physical contact beyond the initial handshake may be inappropriate.

Body Language

Interviewers are often uncomfortable in working with the elderly. This is most obvious in the postures they take during the course of the interview. They walk, talk, and assume rigid sitting postures. Most obvious is what often has been referred to as "hiding behind the clipboard." Even on semistructured interviews, these individuals read directly from their clipboards, rarely look up, and act as if they were automatons.

There is no magical formula for helping someone who is uncomfortable interviewing to feel more at ease. Part of the loosening up of the interviewer's rigidity comes with increasing experience. If the interviewer fears his own aging, for example, and has not examined those feelings, he may never feel comfortable interviewing older adults (Mortimer, 1982). On the other hand, being willing to be open to the experience of learning from one's elders can be sufficiently rewarding and motivating, thereby encouraging the interviewer to feel more at ease with the process. There is a direct relationship between the interviewer's feelings of comfort and the client's.

Showing Respect and Understanding

There is more to the interview process and the development of rapport than is always apparent. The following two case studies illustrate some critical points.

One woman who was being interviewed expressed a great deal of difficulty hearing what was being said to her by the intake workers at an intermediate-care facility. Whenever they asked her a question, she looked back and said, "It's hard for me to hear what you are saying. My hearing aid doesn't help me enough." While she did have a significant hearing loss, medical records suggested that her hearing aid more than adequately compensated for the impairment. Yet she claimed to be unable to hear. A specialist was called in and was asked to attempt to perform an initial psychosocial assessment. At the outset of the conversation, it became clear that, while the woman was complaining about her hearing aid, she was alluding to a completely different issue. The woman was quite nervous and was uncomfortable expressing herself. Having found out from the family that the woman was comfortable in speaking Yiddish, and being reasonably conversant in it, the specialist began to speak in Yiddish. The woman no longer complained about being unable to hear. She was more comfortable and spoke coherently, and the interview proceeded successfully.

Another individual, a male patient in a nursing home, was diagnosed as being aphasic. He was thought to be unable to speak and probably unable to understand what was being said to him. Despite repeated attempts by the staff, the patient was not conversant. Having reviewed his medical and social history, which had come from a hospital, it was determined that his native tongue was Hungarian. The interviewer, who knew a Hungarian folk song, began singing it to him. The client responded rather animatedly and spoke in bursts of Hungarian with only a limited amount of English interspersed. When a staff person was found who was conversant in the man's native tongue, it was determined that the patient was not aphasic but rather had no one with whom to communicate (Salamon, 1984a).

Both of these examples suggest that developing rapport is very much dependent upon the ability to find and respect the level at which the older adult is most comfortable. In a senior citizen center, a place where new clients initially have ambivalent feelings about attending, developing rapport may require indicating that attendance at activities does not necessarily signal that the older adult is growing overly dependent. All it suggests is that the individual likes to find a place to socialize; therefore, the information being solicited at the initial interview is designed to assist the staff in helping in that process.

Sometimes in the process of interviewing, the interviewer will come across an individual who is truly hearing impaired. Often, these individuals will display mild paranoid behaviors. They may express concern that others are plotting behind their backs or are speaking about them "under their breath." Some of these fears may be grounded in reality, and it is important to be able to discern how much is true.

Interviewing individuals with a hearing impairment can be difficult. There are a few techniques that can assist the interviewer in overcoming some of the obvious hardships in communication. To keep the interviewee's attention, physical contact, such as a tap on the arm or back of the hand, interspersed throughout the conversation will direct the client to attend to the interviewer. Speaking slowly, enunciating clearly, and looking directly at the client during questioning all aid in the ability of the client to comprehend.

The interviewer should never scream, but it is fine to speak in a tone of voice slightly above normal. If the client continues to have difficulty in hearing it is not inappropriate to question the client as to which is their better ear, and speak to it. This can be done by using simple sign language, pointing, and so forth. If, after carrying out all of these steps, the client is still unable to understand what is being said, the questions may be written out. In all such situations, it is the interviewer's responsibility to refer the client for a complete audiology exam.

While this discussion of developing rapport touches on many components of the process, it is not exhaustive. If the interviewer uses some of these techniques and couples them with warmth and a true sense of interest, the interview can be a constructive one, performed in an atmosphere of trust.

OUTLINE FOR A GENERAL INTERVIEW

Interviews with the elderly can be performed in a variety of settings and situations and for a variety of purposes. They can be performed as part of a psychiatric assessment; as an intake procedure upon admission to a long-term care facility; as an evaluation for level of entitlement, such as for Supplemental Security Income or food stamps; or for research purposes. Most interviews, however, contain a core of similar items, which tend to fit into five broad categories:

1. A description of the client
2. The substantive reasons for the interview
3. The client's perception of need
4. The client's history, as provided by the client and her or his family
5. A general summary of the interviewer's findings

Description of the Client

The information that must be obtained from the client in all interviews includes a description of the client's age, general appearance, and overall manner. Within these areas, interviewers should be careful to observe the client's behavior; ability to ambulate, walk, get around; and emotional state, especially noting if there are any signs of emotional difficulty such as depression or anxiety.

Interviewers should make note of wheelchair usage or the use of a walker or cane, and how well the client gets around with these. It is also important to take note of any visual or auditory problems the client may have, including noting when the client is wearing thick glasses or a hearing aid.

If the client is not alert but seems depressed or agitated or even if the client appears mildly confused, the interviewer should take note. How well the client is dressed may be an important indicator of need as well as of self-esteem. If the client is wearing old, worn-out clothes but is nevertheless well groomed, this suggests that the client is concerned about the impression she gives to others and wishes to present herself in the best possible light.

How well the client speaks is another important area. The interviewer should observe any difficulties, noting when the client speaks with an accent, is more comfortable speaking a foreign language, has difficulty understanding words, has a history or is presently suffering from aphasia, shows an inability to find the correct words for response, and so forth.

Substantive Reasons for the Interview

Generally referred to as the *presenting problem*, this area includes items such as

1. The primary reason for the referral
2. Where the client was referred from
3. Who made the referral
4. Whether or not the referral suggests that the client had a behavioral problem and was difficult to manage
5. Whether or not there was a sudden change in the client's health status that precipitated the referral

Also of great importance to the interviewer are the client's own feelings regarding the reason for the interview. Often the client can provide information overlooked by the referral source. Items such as the sudden death of a relative or close friend, or some other social or psychological crisis that precipitated a change in the client's lifestyle, may provide information relating to the reason for the interview. The interviewer may develop a more well-rounded picture of the client by attempting to assess this information, generally via an open-ended approach. The client should be allowed and encouraged to express his views freely as to the reason for the referral.

Client's Perception of Need

By pursuing issues related to the presenting problem, the interviewer can follow up on the items perceived as important by the client. Included in this category is an awareness of the client's stated need for the referral and interview. This may include a history of events that occurred at the time of onset of the condition or problems that precipitated the referral.

Occasionally, reactions to losses that preceded the referral may yield information on how well the client is coping with the experience of loss. In addition, individuals' attitudes toward the interview itself and the coping mechanisms they use may subsequently become apparent to the interviewer. Individuals being interviewed as to whether or not they are appropriate candidates to receive, for example, home-delivered meals may indicate a sense of loneliness and depression rather than conveying what was originally viewed as increasing frailty and dependence, the original reason for referral. If such is the case a mental health referral also may be warranted.

If the individual is hospitalized or placed in a long-term care facility such as a nursing home, it is at this stage that the interviewer must examine how well prepared the individual is, both emotionally and physically, for this change. To do this requires careful exploration of the issues related to the client's plans for the future and aspirations for increasing development, and of how realistic these goals are. For example, is it realistic for the person to think he will be able to walk again if all available information suggests otherwise?

An additional, related question is, if and when the client can be discharged from the facility, will she have another place to go? Does the client have a home or apartment? What kind? Is the rent being paid during the period of institutionalization? What about the client's belongings? These items are generally of major concern to the client, and the interviewer should be prepared to deal with them.

Client's History

In addition to the historical items already discussed, the issues in this category require the interviewers' increased attention, as they are more detailed. Items such as choice of religion, importance of religious practice, and educational and employment history all provide valuable insight into the status of the client. The ability to develop friends and the client's own report of her social network are also significant issues related to developing a complete picture of the individual's status.

Older adults often enjoy talking about their early history. Not only is this information interesting from a historical perspective, it also provides information as to the developmental background of the client and his likes and dislikes (Butler, 1975).

Assessing present family history can and should be done by interviewing both the older adult and the family (National Institute of Mental Health, 1979). The assessment should include the strength of the family's ties. While it is often difficult to assess negative family relationships accurately, these issues must be explored, as they can be potential problem areas (Salamon, 1983b). Family can also be important in providing further information as to client's needs, dislikes, habits, and so forth.

One must be careful, however, to distinguish between the reality as expressed by the client and family and wishful thinking on their part. Families often project feelings or interpret life events in ways that are not completely realistic. An interviewer must be wary of families that report that life with their older adult member was always good or always bad.

Summary of the Interview

The interviewer's summary includes an identification of the client's primary problems and any secondary problems or related issues. Often these problems include physical, social, or emotional components or combinations of all three. On occasion, detailed descriptions of the problems encountered in the client can be made after a single interview. If this is the case, the interviewer should be prepared to do so. The summary of findings should also include proposed interventions and reasons for these suggestions.

There are instances when further interviewing is warranted. The interviewer should not view the need for subsequent meetings as a failure of technique. It is, rather, an honest approach to the complexity of working with older adults. If necessary, other interviewers should be asked to help with any additional evaluations. A final summary of findings usually follows a standard format. An example is as follows:

1. *Primary Problem:* Arteriosclerotic heart disease
2. *Secondary Problems:*
   a. Difficulty ambulating
   b. Moderate depression
   c. Restricted social network—few friends, no relatives living nearby.
3. *Suggested Interventions:*
   a. Contact visiting nurse service for physical problem
   b. Order meals on wheels
   c. Recommend mental health evaluation
   d. Institute a home visiting contact

CONTENT AREAS

Within any interview, there is a wide variety of issues, both general and specific, that must be addressed. Depending on the focus and intent of the interview, some of these issues can be examined superfically, while others require a great deal more effort and detail. In this section, we will examine some of the specific content areas that are part of most interviews with older adults. While on the surface some of these points may seem simple and direct, it is rarely the case that a single response is sufficient to evaluate the range of possible answers and their meanings.

Age

A simple question such as "How old are you?" can result in a rather involved discussion. Often responses include, "I am older than you are" or, "I am 21 plus" or, "I don't really want to say." Sometimes evasive answers may indicate a cognitive loss or memory impairment of the client, as evidenced by an inability to remember his own age. A better question to ask is the individual's date of birth. As this involves long-term memory, more directly, it is not as much affected by any disturbance in cognitive functioning. Once the date of birth is obtained, it is appropriate to ask the individual's age. If they can report their date of birth but are unable to compute their age, this may indicate a cognitive impairment.

On occasion individuals may be unable to report their age or even birthdate. This does not always indicate a decline in cognitive ability. Given the nature of birth records of 70, 80, and 90 years ago, it is imperative that the interviewer determine why the client does not remember the date. Often clients will report that no accurate records existed as to the exact birthdate. If the individual immigrated to this country, or if she sought employment while still in her teens, she may have lied or changed her date of birth to fit governmental or employer requirements. She may have reported her age as being older or younger than it actually was, and her "new" age could be the one she permanently adopted from that time on. The interviewer should try to ascertain the most accurate age. This can be done by determining when the individual changed her age, in which direction the change was, and how old she was at the time. It is also important for the interviewer to note the discrepancy between reported age and estimated actual age and the reason for it. Usually, these differences are no more than three to five years in either direction and really do not have a major impact on the interview process.

Another possible cause for not knowing one's exact age may be due to ethnic and cultural background. A Jewish woman said that she was born on the third night of Hanukkah. When her children grew up they selected December fifteenth as being the closest date to her actual birthday. Another woman of Oriental extraction reported that she was born in the third month of the Year of the Monkey. Her children reported her to be in her mid eighties, but she could neither confirm nor deny that.

Age is often seen as a secondary issue in the interview process. Yet, as can be seen from this discussion, it can be used as a means of examining cognitive functioning and also can provide important historical background and thereby insight into the client's life. It can lead to important discussions relating to other issues in the client's life. There are times when clients can give the exact date of their marriages, the births of their children, or the deaths of loved ones. Often these bits of information are extremely important and never should be overlooked.

Living Environment

A case example will make a good illustration of this issue:

A psychologist was once asked to assist in a mental-status evaluation of a woman who did not know where she lived. The initial interviewer had asked the client if she could give her home address. She could not. Feeling uncomfortable in pursuing the interview with this client and convinced that the client was suffering from severe dementia, the psychologist was called in.

This client was seen at an outpatient clinic and was brought to the clinic by her two daughters. The woman was a very charming individual who was well dressed and seemed alert but was simply unable to remember her home address. It appeared that part of the client's inability to remember was her fear of the entire interview process. What started out as a simple request for home-delivered meals resulted in an appointment with a psychologist at an outpatient mental health facility. Above and beyond that, the client's well-intentioned daughters did not tell their mother that she was being taken for a mental-status evaluation.

At the meeting where the mental-status evaluation was performed, the woman was made to feel at ease. She was asked her age, the date, how she came for the evaluation, who the President of the United States was, and so forth—all the necessary components of a standard mental-status evaluation. She responded appropriately to all the questions, indicating that she was alert and not necessarily suffering from dementia or cognitive decline. When she was asked her address, she could not give it. When asked why, her response was, "I never write letters to myself." When asked the addresses of her daughters, she was able to provide both of them accurately, including apartment numbers and zip codes. She then volunteered that she had not been out of her building in five years because the neighborhood had become unsafe. She was afraid of being mugged. When she wanted fresh air, she went out on her terrace.

Following further evaluation, it was concluded that, while the woman was mildly depressed due to her isolation, she was not mentally impaired in any significant manner. While forgetting one's home address can be a sign of organic mental impairment or a developing dementia, this is not always the case. It is important for the interviewer to examine the causes of the forgetting and work to make the client comfortable in providing accurate responses.

A number of questionnaires and surveys require the interviewer to ask respondents if they like their present living environment. The most common response to this question is, "It's my home." This is a perplexing answer, particularly for the researcher who is looking for a yes or no response. The real meaning of the "it's my home" response can be varied. For example, if the individual's home is his own apartment, the response can indicate a fierce sense of independence and desire to maintain the home and hence independence as long as possible. If the individual is residing in a long-term care facility, the response might be said in a tone of helplessness, suggesting that it is not what was wanted, but one has to make the best of one's circumstances.

Perhaps a more accurate question for an interviewer to ask is, "How close to your ideal is your present living environment?" This allows for a discussion of the client's physical and emotional abilities, financial status, and general levels of well-being in relation to his living environment.

Living environment is an issue that is related to other aspects of the client's life as well. Family, friends, general social support, and personality all impact on where people live and how successful they are at maintaining their social well-being (Harbert & Ginsberg, 1979). It is unwise to address the issue of living environment in isolation. It must be examined in context with other items, some of which we now will discuss.

Family

Families can be sources of love, support, and concern, as well as of valuable information in developing personal histories and validating information obtained from the client (National Institute of Mental Health, 1976). On the other hand, much of the family dynamic can be negative and can have a detrimental impact on the client. The interviewer must be careful to comprehend the dynamic before developing a plan for intervention or interceding in any way (Salamon, 1983b).

Manipulation and Guilt. Prior to questioning a family regarding their older adult family member, the interviewer should discuss the need for this procedure with the older adult client. For patients in a nursing home or intermediate health care facility, a great deal of anger may be expressed by the clients toward their families. Angry responses such as, "My family is the reason I am in here" are voiced regularly. While the emotions expressed by the older adult are not always completely negative, they are often indifferent or ambivalent. Responses may highlight a vast expanse of unresolved tensions within the individual and guilt in the family.

Here too, the interviewer must be able to go beyond the obvious anger and determine how much of the expressed emotions are accurate, for both the older adults and their families. Negative reactions to placement may be a verbal attempt to manipulate the family and unconsciously make them feel guilty. The family, in turn, may have had no recourse to institutionalization and may be feeling their own guilt, which is only exacerbated by the older adult's comments.

To relieve tension and avoid confusion, it is appropriate for the interviewer to point out the unwarranted feelings of guilt to the client and the family. This can be done by reiterating the fact that institutionalization was the only viable option and by understanding the pain it caused for all those involved. Without confronting the guilt and manipulation, the interviewer may find it difficult to discern true feelings and obtain accurate responses.

Other responses by institutionalized older adults to questioning by an interviewer regarding the family can seem more positive yet also may express underlying feelings of distress. "I lived my life, now it's their turn" or, "I would only be a burden" are comments that suggest feelings of resignation and a sense of hopelessness and giving up. "The children live out of town, and it's hard to travel" also suggests similar feelings. The interviewer should respond to statements of this nature with a sense of compassion and understanding. One woman, a grandmother whose daughter added two rooms onto her home to allow her mother to be with her and still have a sense of privacy said, "My grandchildren make a lot of noise. They come with friends and it is a tummult." A variety of feelings may be hidden in this comment. Despite the façade of independence for the grandmother, she may feel herself as being forced into a situation of dependence on her daughter. This may be due to her declining physical strength and loss of stamina or the diagnosis and progression of a chronic illness. Her reduced physical capacities are highlighted further by the contrasting youthfulness of her grandchildren. While she dearly loves them, she sees herself as separate and distinct and feels the need to be apart. In this particular case it was determined that, while the daughter had her mother's best interests at heart, she made a mistake in not discussing the plans for a move with her mother. Instead, she renovated the house and presented the two rooms as a *fait accompli*, insisting that her mother had no choice but to move in with her. The mother felt this as an insult to her sense of independence and her hopes of living in her own apartment, even if it required the assistance of a home health aide.

There are those older adults who encourage the loss of their own independence. An older adult mother said of her middle-aged daughter, "I took care of her for many years, now she is taking care of me. It's only right; it's her turn." The daughter said, "I do all of Mom's bookkeeping, shopping, cooking, and cleaning. She's not crippled, though she acts as if she were." Clearly, guilt is being used by both actors in this scene. The mother may be exacting a form of retribution from her daughter, for events that occurred earlier. The daughter, while being obedient and dutiful, may feel pulled in a number of directions—career, family, and now her own mother. This type of role reversal in which the daughter becomes the caretaker for her own mother seems almost always to lead to anger and further guilty feelings.

Worse situations are seen by older individuals who, even though they are being well cared for by a child, will wisely state, "One mother can take care of six children, but six children can never care for one mother."

Interviewers sometimes are misled by statements made by older adults that seem incongruous to reality. When asked about their families, some older adults may respond by saying, "They never call or visit," when in fact they visit regularly and call often. If this is the only statement made that is not reality based, then it suggests that further underlying conflict exists in the older adult, the family, or both. The older adult may want to be more dependent on the family. The family may feel that they have already assumed sufficient responsibility and, for example, visit as often as they possibly can. Guilt and depression may be common in these situations.

Communication and Love. Of course, there are positive expressions made by older adults, about themselves and their families. Sometimes these comments are distinguished more by the way they are said than by the actual words used:

> "My daughter is a famous professor and is doing quite well. They wanted me to move in with them. I thought about it and I realized that, during the day, there would be no one home. Oh, they would hire someone to look out for me while they were away, but I need someone who I could talk to, a friend or a relative. I didn't want to be a burden, so we discussed it and decided that going to a nice nursing home is the best idea."

The expression of good communication and joint decision making indicates that a positive family situation existed in this case.

Interviewers attempt to verify information provided by the client by asking the family to corroborate it. One must not be misled by different emphasis placed on occurrences by different family members. An interesting footnote is that some studies suggest that older adults and their grandchildren tend to report family situations in a more similar fashion than older adults and their children (Harris & Cole, 1980). When the older adults are in their late seventies or eighties, grandchildren may be in their forties and can be considered good sources of information on family dynamics.

Friendships

Social contact, especially having friends with whom to communicate on a regular basis, is important for general well-being and positive mental health. As adults age, they tend to develop a group of friends they have grown close to over many years. These friends are sources of strength and support, both mentally and emotionally. With increasing age, however, one's sphere of friends tends to dwindle. Close friends may move away or begin to die with greater frequency. These losses are major blows to the remaining older adults and may force individuals to reassess the importance they ascribe to friendships. Some individuals react by seeking out new friends, while others spurn all attempts at friendship.

When asked by an interviewer if they had any close friends, residents in a retirement community responded with a variety of comments:

> "I say hello to everybody. I play cards with a group of people and my husband golfs with a few of the men, but we don't have any close friends."
>
> "You can't expect much from these old people, so we are only on polite terms."
>
> "These people are all old and many are sick, not like me, but we all get along very well." [She was 93.]

In the first comment, the respondent implied that it is difficult to have close friends, despite having many things in common with others. She suggested that close friends can be made only in earlier life. Further discussion indicated that she believed that it had been easier to have friends when her children were younger. She was able to share the traumas of early childrearing with individuals who had those things in common with her. There was an underlying denial of a sense of friendship within this woman, which can be viewed as a form of repression and separation. She did not want to make friends, fearing that she might soon lose them.

The other two comments suggest two distinct forms of denial. In the second comment, the individual was distancing himself from his main peer group, in effect denying that he was one of them. There is a refusal on his part to interact with others, suggesting denial of his own needs. In the final comment, the 93-year-old woman indicated a denial of her own aging, but at the same time suggested a healthy interest in interacting with others.

What is most interesting about many comments made by residents of long-term care facilities is that, while these individuals often deny having friends that they are close with, they do have friends with whom they enjoy spending most of their time. These individuals display a clear need for friendship, but at the same time they are fearful of investing any deep emotions or strong feelings in what may realistically be only a temporary closeness. They therefore deny that a relationship exists.

It is important for the interviewer to understand what close friendships are and how they may exist on a variety of levels. Often individuals working with the elderly feel compelled to encourage their clients to have many close friends. While friendship is important for the client's overall well-being, it is also important to recognize realistic fears of loss. Furthermore, the quantity of friends is not what is important, but rather the quality. As a 78-year-old woman in a nursing home put it, "All you need is one close friend."

Often friendships take on a different form in old age than one expects in the younger years. Friendships may be predicated on a card or bingo game. The men who meet in the park and play checkers for two hours may not be seen as having close friendships, because after all it is only a game of checkers, but, nevertheless, on rainy days when the game is interrupted there is a deep feeling of loss. Interviewers must be careful to understand and address these feelings.

Caretakers

Emotional Reactions. Older adults frequently are placed in the care of individuals whom they consider strangers. This can occur both in a facility or institution or even in the older adult's own home. Caretakers, such as home attendants and aides, often provide assistance to the older adult even before a complete interview can be performed. Interviews, therefore, can be tinged with a sense of betrayal and anger for a loss of physical ability or independence. Responses to questions during interviews also may contain elements of fear, guilt, and manipulation. Interviewers have the responsibility to be able to understand the true meaning of what is being said. This can be done only if the underlying meaning can be ascertained.

When asked about how she was getting along with her home attendant, who already had been with her for two weeks, an 82-year-old woman replied, "Even when they don't do something the right way, I just look the other way. I don't want to rock the boat." This response suggests an ambivalent acceptance of dependency and a desire to maintain reasonable cordiality. Yet it also can mask a sense of anger and frustration—anger at the way things are handled, and frustration at being unhealthy and dependent.

Another individual, whose home health aide had been with him for almost a month, responded, "You *have* to accept it." This man suggested that it was difficult for him to accept his dependency and the fact that he needed someone to care for him. His statement was made in a tone of bitterness and clear resentment. While he was not necessarily complaining about his aide's behavior, he was expressing his feelings of depression at his dependency on the aide.

In other instances clients may respond to interview items in specific tones of voice as their means of gaining the attention of the caretaker. Either speaking in whispers or shouting responses may be used as tools by older adult clients to alert caretakers to their feelings toward them. When asked about her feelings of having a home health aide, one respondent raised her voice and said, "It's nice having someone prepare lunch." She then whispered to the interviewer, "But she doesn't make my bed." Another client, during the course of an interview, lowered her voice and asked the interviewer if any of the information she was relating would be told to her caretaker. She expressed the fear that her caretaker might know "too much" about her personal life.

Ethnicity. It is not uncommon for caretakers to be of different ethnic and racial backgrounds than the older adults for whom they are caring. This can cause further difficulty for both the client and the caretaker. One elderly woman of Italian extraction had been mugged and beaten repeatedly in the neighborhood in which she had lived for over 30 years. All the attacks had occured during the last two to three years, during which the cultural makeup of the neighborhood rapidly changed. Following a particularly severe attack, the woman was hospitalized and then placed in a rehabilitation facility where the majority of the woman's caretakers were of the same race as the woman's attackers. In addition to the traumas of the attack and subsequent institutionalization, the woman developed a strong fear of her caretakers. While the fear of attack may have been a reasonable defense when she was living in her old environment, it made her care in the rehabilitation facility more difficult to perform. She was so afraid of her caretakers that she had a hard time letting them take care of her. The interviewer pointed this out to her and also to the caretakers. With time, and with a strong emphasis on caring for her needs shown by the staff, the woman's fear slowly subsided.

Paranoid Tendencies. There are individuals whose fears do not abate. Often the interviewer is confronted with statements such as, "They are stealing from me," "You can't trust them," and "I am missing so many things." The perplexing issue is whether the statements are true and accurate or are paranoid delusions. Often it is not easy to distinguish between the two, and great care should be taken when confronting this issue. It is the interviewer's responsibility in both cases to clarify the fears in the light of past events and present reality and to address them in a manner that alleviates some of the negative emotions. If there is a clear indication that paranoia has developed, a complete mental health evaluation is necessary.

Physical Health

"Ask an older person how they are feeling and you open a Pandora's box." This fear most interviewers have is based in part on reality. The higher rates of chronic illness where both pain and a sense of physical insult can be continuous in older adults may cause many of these individuals to seem unable to deal accurately with their feelings of health and well-being (Furukawa & Shoemaker, 1982). There is increasing indication, though, that older adults accurately describe their health and that their reports of pain are both realistic and truthful (Hickey, 1980; Kopf, Salamon, & Charytan, 1982; Linn & Linn, 1980). What is often difficult for the interviewer is to empathize with the plight of the older adult respondent.

If an older adult says, "It doesn't make sense to complain, but . . .," that almost always indicates that a variety of complaints regarding health and health care are forthcoming. Because the interviewer often represents the health care system, complaints may be taken as a personal insult, resulting in defensiveness. If the interviewee senses the defensiveness, it may be perceived as hostility and as an insult.

Communication and understanding may break down. It is very important for interviewers to say that they understand the pain the older adult feels.

Another common statement made by older-adult health care recipients is, "When you get old, this is what happens." By itself this statement may not indicate anything other than an offhand negativism. If it is coupled with other negative statements, however, it may be one of many indicators of an inability to cope with one's own aging and changes in physical status, or it may reveal a depressive tendency. The interviewer should follow up statements of this nature by asking what the client means.

Older adults tend to report many emotional difficulties in terms of physical problems, and it is important for the interviewer to separate the two. This occurs most frequently if the interviewer is introduced as a doctor. One woman said, "Doctor, I have a terrible headache every morning," but did not report that her headaches were accompanied by crying spells, difficulty sleeping, and a change in her eating habits. Such symptoms would indicate depression, while headaches alone would indicate a wide variety of other neurological or biochemical disturbances. The interviewer must be alert to all symptoms.

Another issue arises when the interviewer is a member of a health care team. The client may indicate a greater degree of need, though not necessarily poorer health. This can be expressed in statements like, "I can walk well with my new cane, but I need so much help with preparing my breakfast." This statement also may suggest a sense of loneliness, which is not a physical need of the client.

Many clients make statements regarding the type of health care they are receiving. Because they experience a great deal of loss as a result of physical changes, these statements may contain much anger and hostility. These feelings are directed toward the health care providers in statements such as, "The doctors don't care" and "You don't get to see the doctor when you need to." One must be able to distinguish between the anger expressed and the truthfulness of this statement. "The doctor never talks to me" is a similar expression of rage and anger. It may indicate that the doctor does not spend a sufficient amount of time with the patient. This occurs often and, when possible, should be addressed by the interviewer.

Statements of this nature also may indicate that the doctor does not tell the older patient what she wants to hear. It is difficult for an individual of any age to be told that her arthritis pain will never completely disappear or that she must stop being as active as she once was. Interviewers must be prepared to deal with the anger and depression expressed by their clients over changes in their physical health, by being caring and sympathetic.

Mental Health

Depression. Throughout the previous discussion, the topic of mental health in older adults has been alluded to. In the elderly, there is an increasing incidence of mental illness. As we discussed in Chapter 3, this may be due to the increasing frequency of depression and dementia (Gatz, Smyer, & Lawton, 1980). Depression often results from the many insults to well-being that older adults must endure, including loss of friends, loss of job, loss of income, and losses due to physical changes. Individuals who are unprepared for these changes often internalize the anger they feel and become isolated, lonely, and eventually depressed. Some of the symptoms of depression include crying spells, changes in sleeping and eating habits, confusion, and increased reports of physical ailments.

The elderly respond well to psychotherapy when their symptoms are due to depression caused by the losses just mentioned. The symptoms of depression, however, may be due to other illness, including metabolic and neurological disease. There are instances when these symptoms may be due to poor nutrition, an unfortunately common situation found in many of the elderly. There are times, though, when the symptoms of depression may be indicative of an even more severe impairment.

Dementia. We saw in Chapter 3 that the common symptoms of dementia include confusion and disorientation, changes in sleeping and eating habits, short-term memory impairments, and even personality changes. In general, there are two types of dementia: those that are irreversible and those that can be cured. The dementias that are reversible are due to a variety of physiological imbalances. To review briefly, the irreversible dementias include those illnesses which cause permanent neurological changes in the brain. Among these are senile dementia of the Alzheimer type and multi-infarct dementia. Until recently it was thought that senility was an inevitable part of aging and due to poor blood circulation in the brain. It is now known that the confusion and loss of memory that are characteristic of senility are a result of a disease process that affects the nerve cells in the brain.

Interviewers occasionally may recognize dementia of this nature by the degree of confusion and disorientation. This recognition alone, however, is not sufficient for a diagnosis. When a diagnosis is made, it is usually done when the disease is in an advanced state and, because other illnesses are expressed with similar symptoms, a diagnosis of Alzheimer's disease is usually a diagnosis of exclusion. A full battery of diagnostic tests must be performed before a definitive diagnosis is made.

Multi-infarct dementia and other disorders caused by cerebrovascular accidents, often referred to as strokes, occasionally cause paralysis, inability to speak (expressive aphasia), and an inability to comprehend the spoken word (receptive aphasia). In instances where the stroke is less obvious, the symptoms may be similar to those of depression.

Using the Interview to Gain Mental Health Information. Major effort has been made to find out more about the causes and treatment of mental illness in the elderly. It is important for the interviewer to gain a great deal of experience in developing a "feel" for the symptoms of these disorders. While any response indicative of disorientation and confusion requires the immediate attention and vigorous intervention of the interviewer, many responses can be differentially diagnosed by their symptoms and severity.

Disorientation refers to an inability to recognize or report accurately the correct time, the correct location, and even aspects of oneself, the person. Disorientation in all three spheres—time, place, and person—often occurs in patients with dementia. Furthermore, individuals with this illness suffer with impairments of short- and intermediate-term memory. Short-term memory is the ability to recall events that happened in the past few seconds, intermediate-term memory involves recall of events that occurred in the past few minutes to hours, and long-term memory refers to things that occurred from several days to many years ago.

While a depressed person will often be able to recall last evening's meal, a person suffering from dementia will have difficulty remembering breakfast. A variety of noninvasive evaluation forms have been designed to assess whether or not dementia exists in an older adult. The most commonly used tools are known as the Face-Hand Test, the Mirror, and the Mental Status Questionnaire (see Table 5–1). To use these instruments requires experience and supervision.

A number of assessment forms have been used in interviews to measure aspects of general happiness in older adults. A variety of scales measure self-reported well-being, happiness, morale, and life satisfaction. There are indications that components of all of these scales correlate well with mental health in the respondents. Individuals who are depressed tend to score lower on some of these measures, while those who are less depressed tend to report higher levels of life satisfaction (Salamon, 1985a).

In addition to depression and the dementias, most of the mental illnesses that occur in the general population also are observed in the elderly. These include anxiety neuroses, phobias, and the major psychoses. In interviewing elderly individuals with suspected mental illness, it is important to take time and not rush the process. It is also critical to develop as detailed a history of the client as possible (Jarner & Verwoerdt, 1975). By proceeding in this fashion, it may be possible to pinpoint situations in the social environment that cause depression. Furthermore, previous test results may be found in a client's history, and these can be compared for changes in the client's profile. By pinpointing these changes, intervention strategies may be begun sooner.

Death

Death is a topic that often is particularly difficult for interviewers to cope with. Older adults, due to their extensive life experiences, have had more experience with death and may have come to better terms with it (Schoenberg et al., 1975). On occasion, however, they are unable to view their own life course in a constructive manner. This is particularly so in institutional and long-term health care settings, which are seen as being debilitative and insulting and places older adults go to to die. Statements such as "They have put me here to die" suggest a strong depressive component and indicate strong anger toward those individuals responsible for the placement of the older adult in the institution, as well as the person's inability to accept his own deteriorating condition.

Denial of one's own mortality may at times be a healthy reaction to a fear of death. Depression also may be considered a reasonable reaction to a fear of impending death (Kübler-Ross, 1979). These reactions often make the interviewer rather uncomfortable, partly due to the interviewer's inability to accept the inevitable. The interviewer may feel compelled to force such clients to accept the inevitable, wrongfully assuming that by doing so they will become better adjusted. This approach, though, may strip clients of their emotional defenses and is disrespectful of clients' ability to work through emotions at their own pace. Compassion and warmth are the most important tools to use in interviews in which death and dying are issues.

SUMMARY

A good interview is an important component in providing care to older adults. There are four key components in developing good interviewing skills:

1. Establishing rapport
2. Eliciting accurate information
3. Asking the appropriate questions
4. Securing sufficient background data

Within each of these components, the interviewer should communicate directly and effectively, clarifying the nature of what is being said and distinguishing the order of importance of the client's problems or needs.

In interviewing older adults it is important to maintain a positive and warm relationship with the client. Regardless of where the interview is being conducted, the interviewer should direct all her attention to the client and what is being said. The interviewer should be sensitive to the client's reactions and also be aware of feelings of discomfort. When these feelings are present, it is important to ascertain why. If the feelings are due to being tired with the length of the interview, it is not inappropriate to cut the interview short and continue at a later time. Pursuing information provided by the client in a supportive manner will yield the most valuable information and most important insights.

Readers who wish to become directly involved in interviewing and assessing older adults should familiarize themselves with the content and use of some of the more widely used assessment formats. These are presented in Table 5–1.

Table 5–1 Formats Commonly Used in Interviews with Older Adults

Physical Functioning and Activities of Daily Living

1. The Index of ADL

   Katz, S., Ford, A. B., Moskowitz, R. W., Jackson, B. A., & Jaffe, M. W. (1963). Studies of illness in the Aged: The index of ADL. A standardized measure of biological and psychosocial function. *Journal of the American Medical Association, 185,* 94 ff.

2. Cornell Medical Index Questionnaire as a measure of health in older people

   Monroe, R. T., Whiskin, F. E., Bonacich, P., & Jewel, W. O., III (1965). *Journal of Gerontology, 20,* 18–22

Table 5–1 *cont.*

3. Functional Health Status

   Rosow, I., & Breslau, N. (1966). A Guttman health scale for the aged. *Journal of Gerontology, 21,* 556–559

Mental Functioning

1. Mental Status Questionnaire and Face-Hands Test

   Kahn, R. L., Goldfarb, A. I., Pollack, M., & Peck, A. (1960). Brief objective measure for the determination of mental status in the aged. *American Journal of Psychiatry, 117,* 326–328

2. Dementia Rating Scale

   Kay, D. W. K. (1977). Epidemiology and identification of brain defecits in the elderly. In C. Eisdorfer & R. O. Friedel (Eds.), *Cognitive and emotional disturbances in the elderly.* Chicago: Year Book Medical Publishers

3. Geriatric Interpersonal Evaluation Scale

   Plutchik, R., Conte, M., & Lieberman, M. (1971). Development of a scale (GIES) for assessment of cognitive and perceptual functioning in geriatric patients. *Journal of the American Geriatric Society, 19,* 614–623

Subjective Well-Being

1. Life Satisfaction Index

   Neugarten, B., Havighurst, R., & Tobin, S. (1961). The measure of life satisfaction. *Journal of Gerontology, 16,* 134–143

2. Philadelphia Geriatric Center Morale Scale

   Lawton, M. P. (1972). Dimensions of morale. In D. Kent, R. Kastenbaum, & S. Sherwood (Eds.), *Research, planning and action for the elderly.* New York: Behavioral Publications

3. Cavan Attitude Inventory

   Cavan, R. S., Burges, E. W., Havinghurst, R. J., & Goldhamer, H. (1949). *Personal adjustment in old age.* Chicago: Science Research Associates

4. The Life Satisfaction in the Elderly Scale

   Salamon, M. J., & Conte, V. A. (1984). *The Salamon-Conte life satisfaction in the elderly scale.* Odessa, FLA: Psychological Assessment Resources

Multidimensional Scales

1. OARS

   Duke University Center for the Study of Aging and Human Development (1979). *Multidimensional functional assessment: The OARS methodology.* Durham, NC: Duke University

2. CARE

   Gurland, B., Kuriansky, J., Sharpe, L., Simon, R., Stiller, D., & Birkett, P. (1977). The comprehensive assessment and referral evaluation—rationale, development and reliability: Part II—A factor analysis. *International Journal of Aging and Human Development, 8,* 9–42

3. PACE

   Jones, E., McNitt, B., & McKnight, E. (1974). *Patient classification for long-term care: User's manual.* DHEW Publication No. HRA 75-3107. Washington, DC: U. S. Government Printing Office

6

Organizing Recreation and Socialization Programs

It is an undisputable fact that recreation programs and socialization activities are good therapy for those who take part in them (McCormack & Whitehead, 1981). Government guidelines for nursing homes and intermediate-care facilities as well as day and nutritional programs for older adults place strong emphasis on providing a variety of daily recreational activities.

Activities programming serves a number of functions beneficial in creating continuity and an interest in living. Not only is recreation highly useful in filling otherwise empty time, but it can help to increase morale, reduce stress and the loneliness associated with depression, and also increase self-esteem (Hastings, 1981). Recreation encourages independence, raises the level of a person's functioning, and enhances the amount of involvement in the community (Macheath, 1984). This helps individuals to overcome their feelings of isolation and loneliness by making them part of a larger social group. This expanded view of self leads to the formation of family-like ties with the larger group, leading to feelings of joy, responsibility, and even occasional disappointment.

In group and social activities, opportunities are created that allow participants to feel useful, needed, and even wanted. Members begin to care more about their personal appearance and to invest greater time in expanding their interests, learning new skills, and experimenting with different hobbies.

A major goal of professional staff in providing programs for older adults is to create, through the activities, an environment that keeps the participating individuals physically and mentally active, helping them to maintain a high emotional and social level for as long as possible. By keeping the body and mind alert, recreation and socialization activities enable participants to take part in daily activities and to cope better with the physical and environmental changes so often associated with aging. When older adults participate in activities, the beneficial effects become evident not only to the staff but also to the communities with which the older adult interacts.

Research has indicated that, given the proper programming, a significant majority of the resident population of any given facility or program will make use of activities and recreational programming (Salamon & Nichol, 1982). It should be noted that participation in activities includes both the core group consisting of those who are actively involved, as well as other individuals who are not totally committed to the group but are nevertheless involved in the group activity process. These two groups can be referred to respectively as *active participants* and *active observers*. Both forms of participation are valid and beneficial for the group members.

A larger variety of activities will meet the needs of a greater percentage of the population exposed to the programming. Very few individuals attend all the activities that are offered at any one site. It is reasonable, therefore, to assume that a proper program of activities has to be tailored to the needs of each individual, not just the needs of the larger group.

Fluctuations in attendance at activities may be due to seasonal variations, changes in staffing patterns, changes in individual health needs, and variations in level of interest. Staff should be sensitive to these fluctuations and be prepared to respond appropriately. One also must bear in mind that the activities program can only be as good as the ingenuity and enthusiasm of the activities program director and staff, but these skills may be learned, developed, and refined.

This chapter presents ideas for organizing recreational activities and socialization programs. These suggestions should be used to expand the range of programming and encourage flexibility in response to each individual's need.

MOTIVATIONAL TECHNIQUES

In this section, we will examine general motivational techniques useful for all activities. Specific motivational techniques for particular activities will be briefly discussed in the next chapter.

Rapport

A trusting relationship is basic to a group leader's success in encouraging participation. The first step, therefore, is to introduce yourself to the participants, as the activities leader, and in turn get to know each person individually. When introducing yourself, give your first and last name and an indication of how you prefer to be called. You also should explain what your role is in the facility. Spend as much time as necessary in developing rapport. Expect that participants also will indicate whether they prefer being called by their first name or the more formal surname. Respect their preference. If they don't specify, always use their surname.

Physical contact is another way to establish a warm and trusting relationship. A warm touch on the shoulder or a firm handshake can be useful in establishing a closer relationship. If a participant is resistant to being touched, they will make you aware of that, and here too their desire should be respected.

Getting Under Way

The second step is to reach out, through the activity, to as many individuals as possible. A music program or a party are both useful activities for achieving this purpose, and they give the program director a chance to observe levels of participation and get individuals interested in recreation as a concept. Although interest questionnaires asking older adults which activities they wish to participate in have been the preferred method of attempting to find out the socialization and recreational interest of individuals, these questionnaires are often unreliable. A more efficient and less time-consuming approach is to begin the activities program as soon as possible. Members of the program should be notified of all the activities via announcements, flyers, and posters on bulletin boards (the use of bulletin boards will be discussed later).

Attendance records should be kept and carefully monitored, especially during the first few weeks of any new program. This allows the activities director to get a better idea of the membership's interests. Attendance should not be the only indication of the successfulness of a program; rather, consistency in attendance should be used as the standard. The attendance record should include the two levels of participation—the active participant and the active observer (or passive participant). Regular attendance and consistent participation on both levels are valid indications of a successful activity. It also would be interesting to note, over time, any crossover of participants from one level to the other.

A decision to discontinue an activity can be based on consistently poor attendance, as indicated by the records. An activity may be discontinued anytime due to lack of interest.

It is impossible at the onset to know all the recreational needs of the membership. As time goes by, it may be necessary to add specific activities to meet the membership's additional needs. There are both formal and informal methods that can be used in determining which activities should be added. The establishment of a Resident Council or Activities Committee are two of the more formal approaches. Encouraging residents to offer suggestions individually, either directly to activities staff or through the use of a suggestion box, is an informal but also very useful approach.

Advertising

When you are satisfied that the needs of individuals are being met by the activities, making the membership aware of the program is the most helpful motivational technique. Frequent public announcement, written information, and personal contact should be a part of the daily routine in encouraging continued participation.

An overzealous activities director may make the mistake of assuming that every member must be involved in programs. Pressure may be placed on individuals to participate in activities in which they have no interest. This has the effect of discouraging participation in general. The activities director should respect each individual's desire, or lack of desire, to participate and should always remember that, given proper programming, the greatest number of individuals will choose to participate.

Recognition

Other motivational techniques are based on giving participants recognition. These techniques include displaying craft items, printing articles written by residents in an inhouse newsletter, and publicity regarding special achievements in local newspapers and the inhouse newsletter.

Snapshots also can be used as a motivating technique. Pictures taken of residents involved in activities and posted where individuals can see them encourage others to share the joy of the experience. Also, people like to see themselves in pictures.

Refreshments

Especially useful as a motivational technique in long-term-care facilities is the scheduling of activities around the mid-afternoon snack. Most individuals partake of the mid-afternoon refreshment and are likely, at the very least, to observe and sometimes actively participate in an activity that occurs at this time. Those activities that allow a great many individuals to participate or are not hampered by the coming and going of group participants, such as social dancing, word games, or music programs, are best suited for this time.

In especially long activities, refreshments can be used to provide additional interest, and they give a means of relaxing during activities that require a higher level of emotional, mental, or physical involvement.

Some Additional Thoughts

Sometimes even the best program falls short because participants are not properly motivated or recognized for their accomplishments. Activities directors should not minimize the importance of motivation and should use their imaginations and be open to new techniques for attracting participants.

Motivational techniques should not be geared only to the participants; visitors should be encouraged to take part as well. They can serve as volunteers to the group leader or can participate along with the group members. Do not lose sight of the fact that having a visitor take part in the activity along with the member is a very powerful motivator. The group members can share their pride and sense of accomplishment along with the visitors.

Program Planning

In the past, social activities group leaders have assumed that people's life experiences made for their hobbies. This assumption led to the belief that if, for example, a person was a seamstress or a tailor they would enjoy sewing or needlepoint for recreational purposes. This, however, is not always the case. Older adults are often eager to get away from their lifelong occupations and look for other areas of interest to occupy their time. Sometimes these people are not sure what activity they might enjoy taking part in. It is for this reason that activities leaders present these individuals with a wide variety of options.

The task of the activities director is to develop as broad-based a recreation program as possible. Being broad based means having at least three or four activities per day, each one chosen from a different category (see the list of activities at the beginning of Chapter 7). A simple beginning could be a morning introductory exercise group, basic arts and crafts group, and a current-events discussion. Once the program has begun, new activities may be added as deemed necessary by the program director, based on responses of the group membership.

In any activity, those who attend regularly are usually the most productive and make up what is commonly known as the core group. This group of individuals has the highest level of interest and will serve to motivate others to participate. Maintaining and expanding this core group should be a concern of the group leader and can be accomplished by offering a "core-group reward," an incentive that provides tangible evidence of achievement and recognition to other participants. For example, in arts and crafts a special sale can be held, the proceeds of which can be used as decided on by the core group. In discussion groups, guest speakers or outings of interest to the participants can serve as core-group rewards. They should be made available to all residents who fulfill the requirements established by the group.

Activity Scheduling

At the beginning of Chapter 7 is a listing that details the four categories of activities. This list should be used as a guide for designing a schedule for your organization. Allow a minimum of 45 minutes in the morning and the same in the afternoon for activities listed under the Discussion Group category. Schedule at least one activity per day from the Physical Activities category, and add further variety from the Board Games and Special Activities categories.

A broad-based program should contain activities that are structured by the team leader and activities that individuals choose to organize on their own. The latter can include card playing, board games, reading, bingo, or any other activity that can take place spontaneously. The group leader's responsibility for these activities is to see that the necessary materials are always available. If pilferage is a problem, a system of signing for materials can be devised.

The Bulletin Board

A bulletin board is an important tool in disseminating information to older adults and thereby serving as a means of motivation. The activities department should have its own bulletin board posted in a site such as the dining area, where there is heavy traffic. In addition to providing a schedule of in-house activities, the bulletin board should contain the following:

1. The location and schedule of activities in nearby senior centers or clubs

2. The location and schedule of religious services, both within and outside the facility
3. The location of convenient shopping areas with stores that offer senior citizen discounts
4. The nearest form of public transportation
5. The location and schedule of movies
6. The location and schedule of programs at libraries, parks, and other local points of interest

It is important for older adults to maintain their ties with the community; if the preceding information is readily available on the bulletin board, this enables them to do so. Nevertheless, it is all secondary to the bulletin board's primary function of containing detailed but brief information on all of the important programs being held in and sponsored by the facility itself.

Length of Activity

Physical exercise activities that require more than a minimum amount of exertion should not exceed one hour. Activities such as dances or walks, which also require physical exertion, usually allow for rest periods and therefore may exceed this one-hour maximum. Except for special events, no one scheduled activity should be held for an entire morning or afternoon.

An optimal amount of time for most activities is between one and two hours. The best guide for length of activity should come from within the participating group. Never lose sight of group members' needs. If you do, motivation will be all the more difficult to maintain.

Use of Volunteers

Often the activities director is faced with a shortage of staff. A good approach for solving this problem is through the use of volunteer recreational aides. These volunteers may be recruited from the community, from staff working in other positions at the facility, or the participants themselves. The latter provides participants with a chance to share their accomplishments with others.

Volunteers may be recruited by contacting local schools, churches, synagogues, and charitable organizations. An advertisement placed in a local newspaper also may attract additional volunteers who are unaffiliated with any of these groups. Visitors to the residence sometimes make the best volunteers. Encouraging them to assist with activities makes for a pleasant visit. These visitors also often are familiar faces and therefore trusted by the residents.

Volunteer recreational aides may be used in two ways: They can be assigned to assist a group leader, or they can run a group of their own. The latter should be done only when they have exhibited sufficient skills and interest. Recreational volunteers who are available to assist on a regular basis should be regarded as recreational staff members and should be treated accordingly. This includes an interview in which skills, interests, and availability are made clear. Like paid staff, these volunteers should be assigned to regularly scheduled activities and should be encouraged to attend staff meetings. When paying positions become available, the volunteers become excellent candidates for these openings.

Volunteers also can be assigned to special events. These events include parties at which volunteers may provide entertainment, useful demonstrations, and special-interest lectures.

Volunteers may be of any age. The opportunity to mix generations should never be overlooked. You should consider programs presented by kindergarten-age children, or friendly visits by people of all ages, as proper use of volunteer groups.

Long-Term Projects

Some individuals have the ability and the desire to maintain an interest in an activity over an extended period of time. In certain instances a long-term project can fulfill the needs of these individuals and is highly motivating. Examples of how this may be applied include the design and creation of an afghan or of a ceramic mosaic, either by an individual or as a group project. Long-term group projects encourage sociability and cooperation among residents. Individuals can take pride in their own personal achievement at the completion of this type of project. Long-term projects also encourage looking toward fulfillment of long-term goals, something older adults often lose sight of.

STAFFING RESPONSIBILITIES

Hours

When discussing a formula for staffing patterns, certain factors need to be considered. Most important is the minimum amount of activity needed to provide a quality program in a facility or institution serving older adults. By way of example, we will take a facility serving 150 to 175 members or participants. To respond to the needs of these individuals a minimum of 50 hours per week of organized activities and staffing is suggested.

Variety

The second element of the formula is variety. A case has been made for the importance of providing programming that meets the individual needs of the entire membership. This can be accomplished with a wide variety of activities within the four categories. The skills that any one group leader can bring to the program will greatly impact on the variety of programming that can be offered. It is reasonable to assume that one staff person cannot enjoy expertise in all areas and that others therefore should be involved.

Budget

Aside from the limitation of any one worker's skills, the budget for recreation and socialization will be established by the administration. The economics of the program are an important consideration.

Keeping three factors in mind—hours, variety, and budget—the following staffing pattern is one possible way of dividing the suggested 50 hours for optimum use. One approach is to have a team of three people working 48 hours between them, along with two program specialists each working one hour per week, thus providing the most effective use of the 50 hours. The breakdown of staff hours would be as follows:

- Team Leader: 25 hours
- Assistant #1: 15 hours
- Assistant #2: 8 hours
- Two specialists: 2 hours (total)

The Team Leader

It is the primary responsibility of the team leader to create an environment that will motivate the membership to pursue their present skills and interests, acquire new skills and interests, and develop relationships, in order to bring hope, joy, and stability into their lives. An additional responsibility of the team leader is to post and maintain an activities schedule. Activities should be held regularly and consistently. Potential program participants should be made aware of activities through verbal announcement, individual contact, and posters on bulletin boards.

The staffing pattern recommended previously provides for a team approach, but a true team approach includes not just paid staff but also volunteers from the community and from within the facility. It is the responsibility of the team leader to oversee the work of these individuals. This includes

1. Consulting with administration on hiring new personnel or accepting new volunteers
2. Helping new personnel to develop warm relationships with group members
3. Assigning personnel to activities in areas in which they exhibit some experience and interest

Once the activity is under way, the team leader should monitor the activity, based on the standards established throughout this chapter. It is worth repeating that consistency is essential. It includes (1) regularity in programming, (2) starting activities on time, and (3) providing the activity in the same place each time.

If we continue to view both the participant and the workers (including volunteers) as part of an extended family, then it could be easy to understand how changes in personnel and the feelings of loss that result may become disruptive to programming. When hiring new personnel, therefore, individuals should be chosen who express an interest and display capability for long-term service. Vacations should be scheduled on a rotating basis so that there is only one person away at any given time.

Activities directors also have a responsibility to the administration; therefore, they must keep records. These records should include not just attendance numbers but the names of individuals and which activities appear to be of interest to them. All of this is easily accomplished by using a sign-in sheet at each activity. (Also recall that the records should include two categories of participation: active and passive.)

After the budget for the program has been established, it is the responsibility of the team leader to stay within that budget. A complete record of both expenditures and income should be maintained and kept current. There should be an accompanying bill for each expenditure.

Team leaders should schedule regular team meetings once every two weeks. All recreation service providers should be encouraged to attend these meetings. They provide a forum at which to discuss relationships with administration, problems with residents, and the sharing of resources. Through the exchange of information these team meetings can be educational and lead to the improvement of skills.

Inservice training is a useful tool in the expansion of the recreation provider's knowledge, adding to the understanding of the physiological, psychological, and social changes that occur as individuals age. Even those who are familiar with this information may not be prepared to deal personally with these changes in their clients. Also, new information on recreational approaches may not be completely understood. It is the responsibility of the team leader to establish a schedule of inservice seminars where professionals teach the recreational staff. Inservice seminars need not necessarily be scheduled within a facility; staff may take advantage of seminars being held at other locations. This also would provide a very useful opportunity for sharing ideas with staff from other facilities.

The Administrator

It is the administrator of any facility providing services to older adults who sets the tone for the care and attention that the participants will receive. Although strapped by fiscal restraints, most administrators take pride in the kind of care they are able to offer their residents or membership. Until recently, however, recreational needs of participants were often addressed in a perfunctory manner. While possibly realizing the importance of recreation, administrators may have felt that providing a recreation program required a great deal of money. Socialization and recreational programming are essential to the maintenance of a healthy outlook on life on the part of older adults. A fully rounded program need not be a drain on the overall operating budget of any facility.

It is the responsibility of administration to provide and encourage activities that will contribute to the health of the participants. This includes

- Establishing a sufficient budget
- Providing an adequate, well-lighted area for activities
- Providing a display area and display case
- Providing storage for crafts projects

To encourage productivity on the part of recreational staff, the administrator should maintain a professional relationship. This would include

- Allowing for the use of the facility's telephone
- Providing space in a filing cabinet
- Giving access to the public address system for activities and related communications

Time allowances should be made for activities directors and group leaders to plan programs and to attend inservice lectures and training seminars: Staff should be paid for this work.

When new recreational staff members are hired, the administrator should consult with the activities director before a final choice is made. Hiring the proper personnel is a major responsibility. The following list should be used as an outline in judging the general qualifications of activities leaders:

1. College-level experience in older-adult recreation or in social services is recommended.
2. In the absence of a college degree, the following minimum requirements should be met:
   a. The applicant should have demonstrable skill in at least two programming areas.
   b. The applicant should be aware of and sympathetic to the needs of older adults.
   c. The applicant should have a true understanding of the value of the recreation program.
3. A warm and outgoing personality is a necessity.
4. The individual can be called upon to work on a regularly scheduled basis and has flexibility in terms of evening and weekend hours.

In addition to the preceding, administrative abilities also may be required. These are useful in terms of budgeting and planning.

THE PHYSICAL PLANT

The design of any facility is a factor that contributes to a sense of comfort and belonging. People tend to congregate where they are most comfortable (McClanahan & Risley, 1975).

Large Groups

Regardless of the actual layout of a particular room, large areas that are centrally located attract people and serve as gathering places. When recreational activities are held in such locations they tend to attract the highest number of group participants. Activities such as arts and crafts, exercise groups, dancing, parties, fundraising, and movies are held most successfully in this type of environment.

Small Groups

Activities such as discussion groups, resident councils, committee meetings, and similar programs requiring mental concentration and emotional involvement are best held in smaller, quieter areas. If such a place does not exist in the building, an acceptable environment can be created by the manipulation of a few small pieces of furniture. Placing a number of chairs in a circle in one portion of the room effectively divides and separates the space. In instances where chairs cannot be moved, a portion of the room can be partitioned off by the strategic placement of a table or sofa. Figure 6–1 presents an example of how this can be achieved. Figure 6–2 shows how a large room can

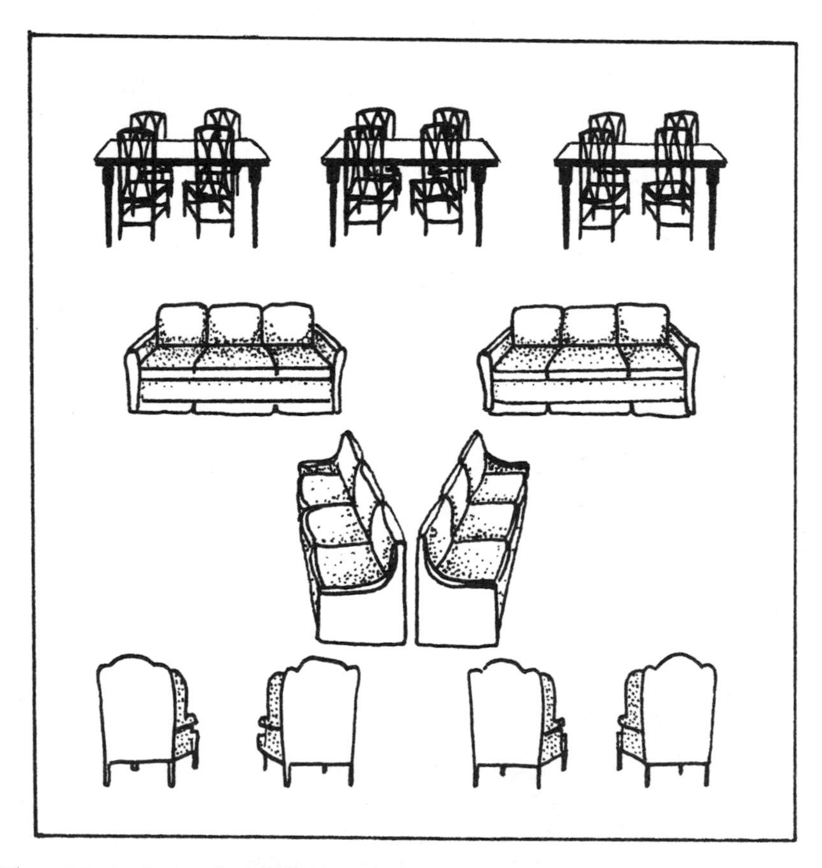

Figure 6–1 Several small-group activity spaces can be created through careful arrangement of tables, chairs, and couches.

be made suitable as a multipurpose room for concurrent large- or small-group activities.

Tables

Certain activities must take place around a table. This is so for arts and crafts, bingo, and a variety of table games. Square tables that seat four and can be placed next to one another, creating a longer, rectangular work and play area, are the most advantageous. Ideally, these tables should have washable, nonglare surfaces and sturdy center bases removing the obstacles that corner legs can create. These tables, when

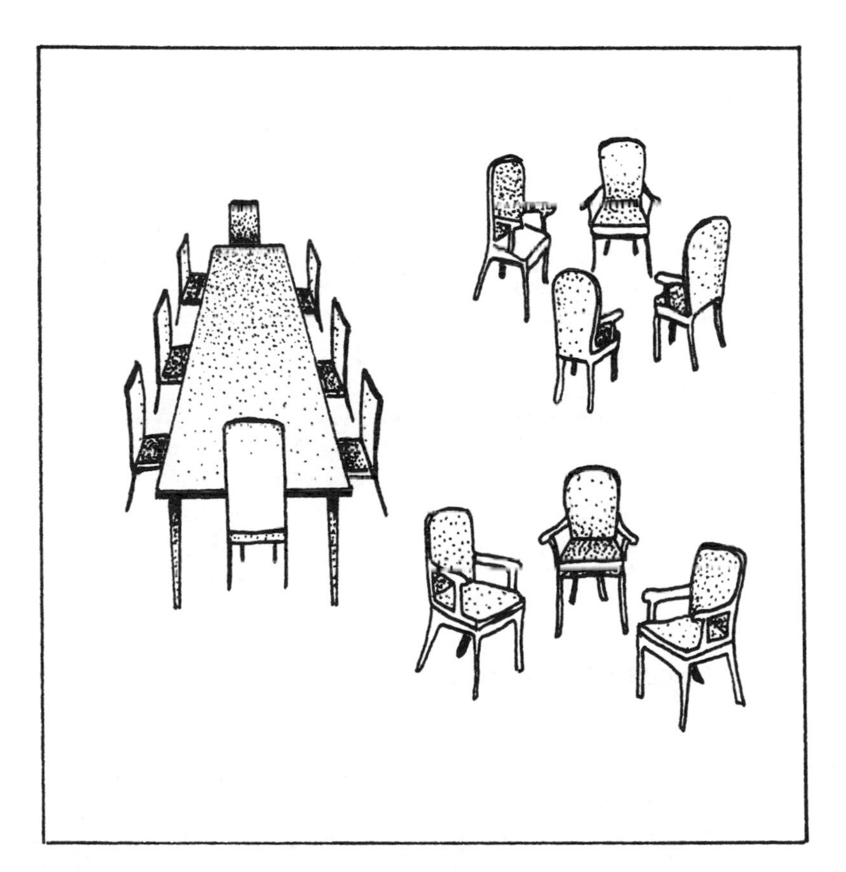

Figure 6–2 Both a large-group area and some small-group areas can be created in the same space, by appropriate arrangement of furniture.

placed together for crafts projects, allow the group leader to work in a more concentrated area. Less time is spent on movement from table to table and more time is spent on the activity.

Where there are only round tables available, a rectangular table can be crated by securely placing a board on top of the round table and covering this board with a washable or disposable tablecloth.

Chairs

Firm chairs with straight backs and side arms are the most appropriate kind of seating for use by elderly group participants. The arms give support when sitting down or rising from the chair. The activities director should be sure to match people with chairs of appropriate height so that uncomfortable seating positions can be avoided. If this cannot be achieved, projects not requiring the use of a table should be substituted. Chairs, like tables, should have washable surfaces.

Lighting

As individuals get older, their visual processes change. Changes in the lens of the eye cause difficulty in distinguishing various shades of color. In addition, the older eye does not adjust as well to background glare. To compensate for these developmental changes, a number of steps should be taken to adjust lighting to make it appropriate for recreational activities. The best visual conditions include a combination of natural, fluorescent, and incandescent light. Work activity areas should make use of this combination whenever possible.

During daylight hours tables may be placed near large windows. Whenever possible, tables should be placed directly beneath ceiling fixtures. In situations where this cannot be accomplished, work areas should be situated so as to provide maximal light with minimal glare and shadow. At no time should fixtures with bare bulbs—or any other bright, unshaded light source—be used. Fluorescent bulbs should be carefully monitored and replaced at the first sign of flickering.

Fixtures

There should be a bulletin board, a large clock, and a calendar at the main activity area and at a strategically located position on all floors of a facility. The calendar will serve the purpose of orienting the individual to time and also will serve to remind the participants of the day's activities. The time of activities can be checked by looking at the bulletin board. Both the calendar and the bulletin board should be designed so that important information is easily seen. Bright colors on neutrally shaded backgrounds, clocks with bold numbers (not roman numerals), type of moderately large size, and nonreflective glass should be used to help in achieving this purpose. Bulletin boards should contain a simple listing of daily activities concisely but tastefully presented.

Public Address System

When announcements are made on public address systems during activities, even discussion groups, they do not necessarily discourage participants in these activities. Indeed, participants sometimes become anxious when activities are held in rooms that are *not* connected to the announcement system, because their fear is that they might not hear a page and therefore miss an important call from a relative or friend. The telephone is the most important link to the outside world, and, while the public address system may seem annoying to an activities leader, it is a comfort to those who participate.

If space allocated for activities is located in an area removed from the general flow of traffic, a greater amount of time should be spent on announcing the activities and guiding participants to them.

PROGRAM RESOURCES

This section provides several lists of basic items needed for various activities programs. As stated throughout this chapter, recreation and socialization activities must be geared not just to the needs of the group but to the needs of the individual as well. These needs may be in flux, so responding to them may require ingenuity. So too with the list of resources. It can be expanded, based upon the needs expressed within the organization in which the resources are employed.

Discussion groups and word-game activities require:

- A portable blackboard
- Chalk and erasers

The following personal grooming items should be available:

- Nail files
- Nail polish

- Nail cleaners
- Wigs
- Combs and brushes
- Mirrors
- Makeup (free samples are often available from cosmetic companies and large department stores)

Arts and crafts activities require

- Yarn, thread, embroidery floss
- Fabric, scissors, pins, sewing and embroidery needles
- Knitting needles, crochet hooks
- Lap looms
- Tiles (mosaic)
- Glue, grout
- Trivets, trays
- Tempera paints, brushes (both wide and narrow)
- Magic markers, crayons
- Drawing paper of varying sizes
- Masking tape
- Stuffing
- Special-interest items such as leather-craft supplies, woodworking supplies, self-hardening clay

Games that are generally used include

- Cards (supply both regular and large face)
- Board games such as Monopoly, chess, checkers, dominoes, Scrabble
- Bingo
- Shuffleboard, adaptable to both tabletop and floor
- Ring toss
- Darts (use velcro darts)
- Softball (supply large-size ball)

Musical programs should have access to

- Record player
- Records (both dancing and listening)
- Song sheets
- Rhythm instruments, including wooden sticks, castanets, maracas, tambourines

Miscellaneous program needs include

- Piano
- Sewing machine
- Sound projector and screen
- Tape recorder
- Amplification system
- Camera
- Bulletin boards
- Large calendars
- Display cases

COMMUNITY RESOURCES

The following are good sources of information on both general and special programs for the aged:

Area Office for the Aging. These offices can provide information on all activities for senior citizens and often hold meetings for those concerned with the problems and needs of the aging. They are a prime contact for information on what is happening in the area and who to contact for additional information.

Area Mental Health Board or Council. These agencies will refer you to organizations providing services to all who need psychosocial rehabilitation activities. They may also provide speakers.

Town or County Department of Parks. These offices may have adult programs on a daily, weekly, seasonal, or holiday schedule; and they may be able to provide recreation specialists for in-home programming or activities at nearby facilities.

Libraries. Special mobile library units often are available to distribute books and large-print reading materials directly to facilities for older adults. They also may offer lectures, films, or records. There may be a mailing list for monthly events. All libraries have books on recreational activities and techniques for enhancing programming.

Local Schools and Colleges. These institutions can provide volunteers who use the facility as a learning environment and bring joy to the participants. All student volunteers should have an advisor in the school who supervises, makes initial visits, and instructs the volunteers.

Organizations and Businesses. Religious organizations, large companies, local merchants, community service organizations, and adult and youth clubs can "adopt" a facility by contributing gifts, volunteers, and transportation and by helping with large mailings, taking over weekends and holidays as recreators or hosts, and inviting residents to their facility.

SUMMARY

In this chapter we have discussed the broad issues in organizing activities for older adults, in particular addressing ourselves to motivation for participation, responsibilities of staff and administration, and the physical setup and resources. In the next chapter we will take a more detailed look at specific activities designed for older adults.

7

Activities Suggestions

The most important step toward a successful recreational and socialization program is to begin to offer activities. At the outset, new programs may not show the usual signs of success. Not having a large turnout, however, does not mean that recreation in general or the activity in particular has been a failure. Rather, this is useful information that may indicate the degree and type of interest of the participants in that particular facility or program. Once programming has begun and a relationship has developed between the staff and participants, changes in activities based on participants' specific needs can be made.

Successful groups are not successful because of the size of the turnout; rather, leaders of successful activities all report the same basic feelings. Most common among these is that they view themselves as being part of a larger group—they often use the word "family." There is a sense of belonging and support that is shared by both the leaders and the participants (Burnside, 1984).

Having achieved unity and a supportive environment, the strength of a group may be directed toward the common goals of the group. These goals could be as simple as enjoying oneself during a social dancing hour, or they can be as complex as solving individual problems, for example, overcoming feelings of isolation and loneliness. Helping individuals successfully to realize a group's goals, such as learning a simple crafts project, is an element toward which all activities leaders should work. A group is made up of individuals, however, and group leaders must work with each individual to achieve group success.

When a new activity is being introduced, it is important that participation should not be frustrated by complicated instructions. Start with relatively easy tasks. A couple of suggestions are (1) a simple craft project such as decorating a small, empty soda can to be used as a catchall for personal items and (2) a simple circle dance that involves walking first in one direction and then the other, followed by hand clapping, and then repeating this pattern until the record is over.

It is a good idea to interrelate the variety of activities offered at each site. This will broaden the interest of the participants, who might otherwise limit themselves to just one or two activities. For example, if a dance is planned, the decorations could easily be made by the crafts group. This type of program planning helps to bring groups with divergent interests together by creating a common goal.

FOUR MAJOR ACTIVITIES CATEGORIES

The following lists of activities give some examples of the kinds of programming that do not require a great deal of monetary investment but are frequently successful. Activities should be tailored to the needs of the members of each program. Group activities can be divided into four major categories or areas, which will be outlined first and then discussed in detail.

1. *Discussion Groups*. These are activities in which no excessive physical output is necessary but where mental concentration and emotional involvement are needed.
   - Current events and citizenship groups
   - Religious services and Bible study groups
   - Resident council
   - Sing-alongs
   - Choral and drama groups
   - Literature and poetry groups
   - Discussion and debate groups
   - Complicated arts and crafts projects
   - Clubs and committees
   - Lectures
   - Educational classes
2. *Physical Activities*. These require more than a minimal physical output on the part of the participant.
   - Exercise, including some forms of physical therapy, aerobics, tai-chi, and so forth
   - Social dancing, such as square dancing, ethnic dancing, and the like
   - Walks
   - Trips, including day and overnight outings to sites of interest

Sports, such as shuffleboard, ball toss, and so on
Setting up for activities (moving furniture, setting out supplies, decorating for parties)

3. *Board Games.* These activities do not require a great deal of physical, mental, or emotional involvement.
   Bingo
   Card and table games
4. *Miscellaneous Other Activities.* These activities do not fit comfortably into the other three categories but are generally socially motivating and should be part of a comprehensive recreational program.
   Parties
   In-room activities
   Cooking and baking
   Special events
   Facility newspaper
   Service projects
   Movies
   Lobby games
   Simple crafts projects

Discussion Groups

Discussion groups are extremely useful in countering feelings of isolation (Burnside, 1984; Kartman, 1979). Participants have the chance to communicate with and develop an awareness of the feelings and thoughts of the others. There are many different kinds of discussion groups, all of which are enjoyable to older adults. By holding intellectually stimulating conversations with others, discussion groups help individuals to achieve a sense of identity and accomplishment (Stabler, 1981).

Discussion topics relating to the participants' life experiences create an atmosphere of sharing and enable group members to view one another in a broader, more fully rounded and healthy fashion. They also provide an important boost to an individual's sense of self-esteem.

Problem solving is another area to which a discussion group can address itself. In this type of group, participants share their concerns and help one another by being supportive, caring, and understanding of one another.

Current events discussions that deal with issues taken from the daily newspaper are useful tools in reality orientation. By reestablishing a link with events that occur in the present, a frame of reference and a concern for today are created (Merrill, 1974).

Techniques. To begin a discussion group, announce the formation of the group three to five weeks before its inception. Do this at one of the other, more popular activities that take place in the facility or program. Next, put up posters around the facility and continue to make weekly announcements of the existence or meeting of the discussion group. Posters should be printed in large type, colorful, eye catching, and easy to read. Use pictures if possible, either drawn or cut out from magazines.

The discussion group should take place using either a round table or chairs set up in a circle. This clearly indicates that all group participants have equal input. A set of rules for participation should be stated at the first session, and the participants should be reminded of them, in capsule form, as needed at following sessions. The standard rules for a group discussion are:

- Only one person can speak at a time.
- When one person speaks, everyone in the group should listen to that individual.
- Others may comment or disagree, in turn, one at a time.

There is nothing wrong with reminding group members during the discussion that the rules still apply. This should *not* be done in a condescending or reprimanding tone; rather, the leader should say, for example, "It is not possible to hear anybody well when more than one person is talking."

If the group leader finds that one particular individual seems to be controlling the conversation, then that leader, whose role is that of facilitator, may say, "Thank you for your insight" or, "We appreciate you sharing your thoughts with us, but I think it is time we heard from some of the others in the group." Often a touch on the hand by the group leader may stop a controlling speaker or encourage a quiet group member to begin contributing. Another way to encourage participation by passive group members is to start a discussion wherein every member of the group has to respond. This way, as the people in the circle respond, the quiet people will not feel singled out; in fact, they may welcome the opportunity and begin to feel quite comfortable in responding.

The optimum size for a discussion group is between 12 and 18 participants. If more people than that wish to join, it might be best to make two groups.

Discussion-group leaders should always be aware of the perimeter of the group. Those people who do not wish to sit within the circle but enjoy listening to the discussion and sit on the outside of the circle are passive participants. Sometimes (and it should be a goal) a passive participant becomes an active participant.

There is only one basic requirement for a discussion group leader, and that is to be prepared—do some research and have a knowledge of the topics that will be discussed. This means that, for example, the discussion leader must read a newspaper before having a current-events discussion. Some possible sources for discussion topics are television and radio shows, movies, short stories, poetry, magazines, and books.

A discussion-group leader benefits along with the participants by gaining further insights into the residents' personality and opinions. The leader also has the unique opportunity of experiencing, in a very personal way, important events of the past that the discussants may bring up.

Political Action Groups. It is important that the aged continue to have the opportunity to exercise their rights as citizens and to take an active role in local, state, and national issues. A natural outgrowth of a regularly scheduled current-events discussion group would be specific activities related to political action. One suggestion for an activity relating to political action is voting. Participants of programs for the elderly may choose to vote at their local polling place or cast absentee ballots. Your local chapter of the League of Women Voters can supply you with the necessary information to implement registration and voting.

Social action around issues related to older adults is another political action activity. Increases in Social Security benefits, expanded medical coverage, or other entitlements that directly affect group participants are topics to which a political action group can address itself effectively.

Arranging for guest speakers and posting notices with the dates and times of relevant television and radio programs also will keep the participants informed of the issues. Those who choose to will feel secure that they are casting an intelligent vote. One activity that heightens interest in voting is to conduct a straw poll by making a list of likely candidates for any given office and having group participants vote for their favored candidate. It is interesting to repeat the straw poll periodically, to see if the program reflects the opinions of the general population.

Resident Council. Active participants in political action activities often become candidates for a resident council, which as one of its functions addresses itself to social action issues within a particular facility or program. A successful resident council can be established by using the guidelines in *Establishing Resident Councils* prepared by Barbara M. Silverstone (1974). In it, she makes the following statement of the goals and operation of a resident council:

> A resident council is an organization of the persons living in a home, nursing home, or apartment house for the elderly. All residents of the facility automatically become members of the council. A council operates independently, but in partnership with the board of directors, administration and staff of the institution. Officers and representatives of the council are democratically elected and activities are governed by democratically adopted by-laws, consistent in their provisions with the by-laws of the institution or home.

The establishment of a resident council is one of the most effective forums for building understanding and communication between the participants or residents and staff.

In one case example the food committee of the resident council in an adult day program requested that desserts at noontime meals be more varied. When they discussed the problem with the administration and the cook at a council meeting, the staff expressed no objection to varying the dessert choices but explained that when they did so the other participants requested the dessert they most frequently served. The food committee brought this information to the participants, and the problem was resolved successfully by setting up an alternative schedule with options for dessert.

In another example a request from the resident council in an intermediate-care facility suggested more frequent arts and crafts sessions. The activities director explained that there was limited interest in crafts sessions and that it would be unwise to divert resources from other activities to accommodate a few at the expense of many. The compromise was to have available, as an unstructured activity, crafts materials that could be used by those desiring to work independently.

Religious Activities. Religious activities have a very special place in the lives of many older adults. Aside from adding to their spiritual strength, religious services recognize the residents' need for continuity with important traditions and the past. This is an important factor in the adjustment process that takes place in older age. There is a continuity in feelings of being useful and needed by the larger religious group, as well as the continuity of a sense of dignity and pride and feelings of warmth and love within the greater religious movement. These feelings can serve to encourage growth both emotionally and educationally, leading to greater feelings of self-worth throughout the life course.

Religious activity groups should be geared not only toward the group as a whole, but, as mentioned before, toward the needs of the individuals who take part in the activities. Participants should be able to find religious services that fit closely with their own spiritual needs. It is the responsibility of the activities director to get a list of the residents who wish to take part in services. That list should then be expanded to include the residents' faith, commitment to the faith, and type of services these individuals would be willing to attend. Arrangements should be made to meet the needs of all these individuals. Rooms should be set aside and regular times reserved for religious programming.

Often it is difficult to meet all the spiritual needs of all the residents. In such cases, arrangements can easily be made with local churches and synagogues. These houses of worship might supply a religious leader who would attend the program regularly and visit with individuals of that denomination. Oftentimes houses of worship will supply prayer books and other items needed for religious services in the institution. If arrangements cannot be made to have services in the facility, houses of worship are generally eager to help make arrangements so that participants of the institution might find transportation to services held at the local church or synagogue.

Religious services and other religious activities provide a much-needed form of spiritual therapy. These can include Bible discussion, religious music, religious instruction, and religious arts and crafts projects. These programs offer insights to religion, God, and the meaning of life. In this way, it becomes an uplifting experience, something to which participants look forward and in which they take great pride.

Musical Programs. Some of the most popular activities scheduled by activities staff are those involving music. These types of programs have broad appeal. Members benefit from either direct participation or from listening and observing. Since musical tastes vary, many different types of musical activities can be held successfully. One of the simplest programs to perform and one that is also easy to organize is a sing-along. Familiar songs from the past allow for the greatest amount of involvement. Song sheets in large print should be distributed to each individual. Live musical accompaniment, provided by the group leader or a volunteer, is most desirable. Participants can request their favorites so that no particular order need be followed. A less desirable but no less appropriate alternative is to hold a sing-along to recorded music. It is also possible to have a community sing without musical accompaniment.

Another program, involving recorded music, is listening to show albums. Records can be either purchased, borrowed from a library, or donated. The group leader should first explain the story line of the play. When the record is played, residents can be encouraged to sing or hum the more familiar tunes. The members can then discuss the story line and offer their opinions on the major events of the show. If the album is too long for one session, two or three sessions can be held to listen to it. A review of the past sessions should be given as a reminder for those who attended and to bring new participants up to date.

Music clubs can be formed for those who have a preference for classical music, opera, religious music, or foreign-language or ethnic songs.

A rhythm band using instruments such as triangles, bells, rhythm sticks, small drums, maracas, and tambourines is an excellent suggestion for entertainment at parties or as a musical program. Volunteer musicians or recordings of songs with a lively beat provide the best type of background for a rhythm band. Demonstrate each instrument and allow the participants to select the ones most appealing to them.

Give individual residents who express interest the opportunity to perform. Spontaneous performances or a more structured activity such as a talent show should be encouraged. Groups or residents also can be organized to form a choral group, orchestra, or band. Regular rehearsals should be held, and the groups can perform both within the program and for outside organizations and groups.

Arts and Crafts. Arts and crafts activities satisfy a need for creativity and self-expression. They involve the participants both physically and mentally. They also help heighten self-esteem when finished items are displayed and admired by all who see them. Arts and crafts activities can be as varied as the materials on hand and the imagination of the group leader and participants (Gould & Gould, 1971). Consider the skills, interests, and needs of the members when planning for these activities.

- Some individuals with limited interest or capabilities might prefer a simple project that can be completed in a short period of time.
- Others may be willing to work on more complicated, long-term projects.
- There also may be times when a participant is skilled in a medium in which only she can work.

Whenever possible, opportunities should be offered in all of these categories. There should be a chance for the skilled to pursue existing interests, and there should be instruction for those who are unskilled but are interested in learning.

Materials for arts and crafts projects can be acquired in a number of different ways. Direct purchases can be made, based on both budgetary restraints and their continued use by the members. Letters can be posted requesting donations from visitors. Another way of obtaining funds for materials is to produce items for sale. For example, participants can make two items, one to be kept by the member and the other to be sold for an amount that will cover the cost of the raw materials for both items. The sale of finished projects can be ongoing or can take place at periodic craft sales. If there is money available after all materials and supplies are purchased, these funds can be used for a group reward.

The following are general rules for all arts and crafts projects:

1. Use an area that is well lit.
2. If the project will create dust or a strong odor, be sure the area is well ventilated.
3. The leader should be familiar with the steps necessary to complete each project.
4. When possible, have a sample of the completed project available.
5. Adapt the project so that members with limited capabilities can participate.
6. Clearly label all unfinished projects so they can be returned to and be completed by the participants.
7. Keep instructions clear and easy to follow.
8. Be patient and offer encouragement when needed.

Some possible suggestions for crafts projects are

1. Greeting cards for use at birthday parties or as get-well cards.
2. Identification cards to be used by volunteers or participants on outings or trips.
3. Decorations for special events.
4. Tissue-paper flowers to be presented to those participants receiving special recognition (birthday party, service, achievement, and so forth).
5. Aprons for volunteers serving refreshments.
6. Knitting and crocheting (scarves, hats, booties, afghans).

7. Sewing and embroidery (handkerchiefs, pot holders, pin cushions, sun hats, tote bags, stuffed animals, mending).
8. Wool crafts (rug hooking, pictures, wool winding, dust mops).
9. Copper crafts (small pictures, jewelry).
10. Leather crafts (lanyuard, book marks, comb holders, key cases).
11. Clay crafts (animals, planters, bowls, flat decorated plates).
12. Mosaic tile (creating designs for trivets, trays, ashtrays, and empty boxes).

There are many projects that can be made from leftover supplies or materials easily acquired either at low cost or for free. Buttons, shells, dried beans, pasta, small stones, pictures from magazines or old greeting cards, or anything else on hand may all be used to decorate empty boxes, cannisters, bottles, or jars. These items make useful containers or decorations. Collages, plaques, and other wall hangings also can be made from such materials. Scraps of fabric can be used as stuffing or for patchwork projects (Kay, 1977).

Books, magazines, pattern companies, and the skills of the activities director, participants, and volunteers are all excellent resources for arts and crafts project ideas.

Physical Activities

It has often been said that the aged are "out of touch" with their bodies and their physical feelings. They don't feel in control of their bodies. Even those who at one time led active, physically productive lives exhibit patterns of weakness, lethargy, and even laziness. The purposes of a physical fitness group are:

1. To develop bodily awareness
2. To develop awareness of the importance and value of entering into an exercise program
3. To encourage people to exercise to ward off pain due to lack of mobility and motion
4. To emphasize the importance of walking and keeping physically fit
5. To keep muscles flexible and strong, as weakness and stiffness of muscles can make anyone feel old
6. To stimulate the entire circulatory system
7. To sharpen the mind
8. To avert depression
9. To cultivate the experiences of better sense of self and feelings of well-being

10. To educate the administration and staff of the facility to the value of the program and to gain their cooperation in encouraging the participation of the residents

The quality and nature of the relationship between group leaders and participants will have an important effect on the development of the physical fitness group. Good rapport with participants is of primary importance in motivating them to participate and discover their capacities. The following techniques are useful in establishing a successful and enjoyable group:

1. Encourage yourself and members to feel at ease. There should never be a competitive atmosphere among group participants.
2. Show an interest in each individual by giving everyone some recognition.
3. Show support, approval, and confidence to group members.
4. Encourage participants to practice at home, on days when the group does not meet.
5. Cultivate good communication, as it will enhance the value of the program. Encourage yourself and others to speak up and spread the joyous feeling.

A standard exercise program should consist of three basic parts: warming up, peak work, and cooling off. The exercise portion of a physical fitness program should start with 15 minutes of exercises, built up slowly to a program of no more than 45 minutes of exercises. When you have reached the 45-minute maximum, the class should be structured somewhat as follows:

- 10 minutes of breathing or other warm-up techniques
- 10 minutes of chair exercises to prepare for the more strenuous activities
- 10 minutes of standing exercises, which also can be done seated by those who cannot stand and exercise
- 5 minutes of relaxation to begin the cooling off
- 10 minutes of related discussion to encourage generalization of the sense of well-being

Breathing Techniques. The complete and proper breathing techniques should be emphasized. One should breathe in through one's nose, filling the lungs down to the lower lobes, with the stomach pushing outward. The air should be allowed to flow in, filling the remainder of the lung area. Exhaling should be done slowly, blowing the air out gently through the mouth. This should be repeated three or four times. It increases the oxygen intake and also serves to relax the body.

Chair Exercises. The following is a list of chair, or seated, exercises. Choose a few to begin with and add more as the group progresses. The language is appropriate for use by the leader with the group.

1. Point and flex your toes with your legs stretched forward.
2. Scissors, up and down. Keep your knees straight and your legs elevated. Take small and large kicks in any sequence.
3. Scissors, crossing horizontally, opening and then crossing your legs (cross–open–cross–open).
4. With your legs stretched forward, and arms stretched forward, roll your ankles and wrists in each direction, first clockwise, then counterclockwise. Ten times in each direction.
5. Click your heels together. Open your legs apart widely between each click.
6. Click your toes together. Open your legs apart widely between each click.
7. Bend your knees in toward your chest, alternating legs. Hold the knee in position near your chest, with hands around the knees for a count of 10.
8. Hold your right leg under your right knee, with the right foot lifted above the floor. Roll your knee around clockwise (about 10 times) and then counterclockwise (about 10 times). Do the same procedure with your left leg. Repeat two or three times.
9. With your hands tucked in back of your head and your elbows outstretched, stretch to one side, reaching your elbow toward the seat of the chair—straighten—then stretch to the other side, reaching your elbow toward the seat. Repeat five to 10 times (depending on the physical condition of group members).
10. With your hands tucked in back of head and your elbows out, twist at the waist with the entire upper portion of your body, looking back at your elbow, and then straighten. Repeat five to 10 times (again depending on physical condition of group members).
11. Alternate leg kicks, kicking each leg up and down (can be done while raising arms simultaneously).
12. Alternate leg kicks, kicking each leg out to the side (also can be done while raising arms simultaneously).

13. With your arms stretched forward and your elbows straight and fists clenched, twist your wrists from side to side as you slowly raise your arms above your head, then out to the side, then forward again. Repeat two or three times.

14. Open and close your hands, palms facing the ground, stretching your fingers as you do. Keep your elbows straight. Repeat with the palms facing upward. Start slowly and then progress more rapidly. Repeat until you start getting tired.

15. Neck rolls: Sit comfortably in the chair, keeping your spine erect and your hands at rest on your knees. Now, lower your chin to your chest. Lower your right ear to your right shoulder. Drop your head back gently. Lower your left ear toward your left shoulder. Do not strain. Continue from one position to the next in a gentle, circular fashion, repeating three times. Then reverse the direction and repeat the sequence.

Standing Exercises. These exercises should consist mainly of stretching. Here, too, they are written in language that may be used by the group leader. For those older-adult participants who have difficulty standing, the activities can be adapted for sitting.

1. Hold your arms above your head, elbows straight. Reach toward the ceiling. Fingertips should be stretched upwards. Repeat 10 times.

2. Keep your arms above your head, lock your thumbs together, and keep your elbows straight. Twist left at the waist and look under your right arm, then straighten. Twist right at the waist and look under your left arm, then straighten. Repeat two or three times to each side.

3. Stand tall and erect. Interlock your hands behind your back, with elbows straight. Inhale as you raise your arms in back of you, keeping your hands interlocked. Hold your interlocked hands at their highest point and exhale as you stretch just a little bit more. Hold for a count of five, then release slowly. Repeat two or three times.

4. Stand with your legs apart, arms outstretched at shoulder level. Keep your elbows straight. Inhale. Exhale as you bend to the right slide your right hand down the side of your right leg. Looking straight forward, hold that position (count anywhere between five or ten, depending on the physical condition of group members). Inhale as you rise to a standing position. Exhale as you repeat the procedure on your left side. Repeat two or three times to each side.

5. Stand with your arms outstretched at shoulder level. Inhale. Exhale as you slowly stretch forward, reaching diagonally across with your right hand pointed toward your left ankle (or wherever hand can

reach on left leg). Hold the position, breathing in and out through your nose. Inhale as you rise to a standing position. Exhale, bowing forward and reaching diagonally across with your left hand toward your right ankle (or wherever hand can reach on right leg). Hold that position, breathing in and out through your nose. Repeat one to three times (depending on the physical condition of group members).

Music can and should be used in conjunction with the exercise program. Any music with a heavy beat played at a moderate volume is generally appropriate and encourages more rapid movement. It is also an excellent mood elevator.

Dance. Dancing is an activity that, for most people, brings back happy memories and suggests future happy occasions. It is often a time for dressing up and celebrating. On the occasions when dance is the main activity, people touch, talk, look at each other, and feel closer to one another (Caplow-Lindner, Harpaz, & Samberg, 1979).

Visitors to programs for older adults often visit when a dance group is in session. This is probably so because the visitors find the participants in a happy mood, and the visitors themselves enjoy dancing. Group leaders should take advantage of this and invite visitors to participate. In addition, the participation of nurses, aides, activity directors, cooks, and office, medical, and cleaning staff should be encouraged. The group participants and their visitors can relax and enjoy each other, and staff are seen in a more human light.

Dance instructors should dress in brightly colored clothes. This helps to set a positive mood for the activity. Group leaders should have a knowledge of many different types of dances and be sufficiently skilled to adapt them to the needs of their special population. Dances that are long-time favorites, such as the two-step, and favorites of today, such as disco, should be part of the dance program.

Dance is generally a very well-attended activity; therefore, a large, well-lighted room, free of obstacles, with chairs set around the perimeter makes for the ideal setting. When such space is unavailable, any room where there is enough space for dancing will do. Use a record player that provides a clear sound that is loud enough for all to hear. Even before the dancing begins, play gay, melodic music. It helps to alert everyone to the upcoming activity. The dance group should begin with an exchange of warm, friendly greetings. The leader should reassure participants by saying, "If you can walk, you can dance. Dancing is no more than walking to music."

The first dance should be uncomplicated and act as a warm-up. Start with an easy line or circle dance. Use movements such as walking, turning, swaying, clapping, and stepping in place. There should be no pressure to dance, but everyone in the group should be involved. Ask participants to clap their hands and tap their feet to the music and to create their own steps in time to the music. Allow time for both group dancing and one-to-one dancing. Vary the tempo, and allow sufficient time for resting. During rest periods continue to play the music and engage in discussion with the group members. Use suggestions from the participants, or even some of their own records, as this adds to the feeling of joy by bringing back pleasant memories.

It is a good idea to close the session with the same dance the group began with. Participants will then have a sense of closure and a feeling of accomplishment.

Dancing is a very warm and loving way to fulfill the physical and emotional needs of older adults. Remember, though, not to make it too strenuous. Dance groups should last between 45 minutes and one hour and have at least two five-minute rest periods.

Outings and Trips. Outings are an important way for residents of facilities for the aged to maintain contact with the outside world. When planning a trip or an outing, several important points must be addressed, including the following:

1. Is the destination near or far? What are the scheduled times of arrival and departure?
2. Can the vehicle park near the entrances? How far a walk is it from the vehicle to the building?
3. Are toilet facilities convenient? Is there a toilet on the bus or train?
4. If you are taking along meals, make the necessary arrangements with the kitchen staff well in advance of your trip.
5. In the case of a show, where are the seats? Are they near enough to the stage for participants to be able to see and hear the actors?
6. Are there enough staff or volunteers to accompany participants?
7. Each participant should have visible identification, with name, address, and telephone number.
8. If you will be late for dinner, make arrangements with the kitchen staff.
9. Accept as participants only those individuals who can handle this particular outing.
10. Leave with staff at the facility a detailed itinerary and the names of participants and staff who are taking part in the outing.
11. If needed, have the participants sign consent slips.
12. Always bring a snack, in the event you get caught in traffic.

Outings that are planned by the participants themselves are usually the most successful. Participants should be given choices for outings, from which they can select. Some of the many possibilities include performances at local schools, concerts, shopping trips, museums, movies, theaters, other senior centers, and boat rides.

Miscellaneous Other Activities

Special Events. Special events should be just what the name implies—special. They are events that occur less frequently than do regularly scheduled activities and are organized around a unique theme. Special events can be held as often as a monthly birthday party or as infrequently as once a year (Barnes & Shore, 1977). Group members look forward to these special occasions, and they present an opportunity for involving many individuals in the planning and carrying out of the event.

A theme should be agreed upon well in advance of the scheduled date so that enough time is allowed to complete all the necessary arrangements. Appropriate decorations can be designed and made by crafts groups. If entertainment is to be provided through an outside source, make sure the date is available and reserved. When planning refreshments, keep in mind those people on special diets. If refreshments are to be provided by the facility, coordinate with the kitchen staff. Be sure you have enough help from both staff and volunteers. Publicize the event with special posters, and send invitations to families and friends if the group members agree. If the event is in honor of an individual or a group of people, have them seated where they can be seen and congratulated by the other participants. A paper corsage or boutonniere also will make those being recognized feel special.

Some suggestions for special events include birthday parties, holiday celebrations, fashion shows, volunteer recognition, ethnic themes, and a Las Vegas night.

Facility Newspaper. There are a number of very important reasons to print an in-house newspaper:

- Upcoming activities can be publicized.
- Special events in the lives of the participants can be noted.
- Individual or group achievements can be applauded.
- Participants are provided with another medium through which opinions and ideas can be expressed.
- Members can see their own creative writing efforts in print.

The subjects can be as varied as the contributions of the residents allow them to be. Current events, book reviews, poetry written by members and staff, recipes, past remembrances, and group-member profiles are just some of the possibilities.

This is one project in which participants can assume total responsibility, once enough interest has been generated. Recruit participants with some skills in writing or illustrating, along with those who will serve as reporters, distributors, and typists. When there are enough volunteers to form a newspaper committee, a meeting should be scheduled. Initial assignments, such as the process for selecting a name, cover design, and articles, should be discussed. The newspaper should be typed in large print (e.g., IBM Orator ball) to enhance its legibility. Copies should be distributed to all staff and participants, with extra copies printed for visitors. There also may be times when a group member will want extra copies for family and friends.

A facility's newspaper reflects the capabilities, attitudes, and concerns of its members. It can contain as little or as much information as agreed upon by the committee. The following questionnaire is useful in gathering information for the newspaper

The Sunshine House Good News

We want your "good news" to print in the newspaper that is coming out very soon.

Your name ____________________

Good news: Do you know of someone who recently recovered from an illness? How about some good news from your family? ____________________

____

Births ____________________

Marriages ____________________

Bar Mitzvah ____________________

School Graduation ____________________

Give your family members' names ____________________

Anniversaries ____________________

Any especially nice memories you would like to share? ____________________

____

Give us some good news about the weather? ____________________

____

Good thoughts? ____________________

____

How about some good, pleasant gossip? ____________________

____

Movies. The viewing of movies in a facility has been shown repeatedly to be one of the most popular group activities. Movies attract a large number of individuals because they are a form of entertainment to which many of the group members have gone throughout their lives, so they are welcomed for the sense of continuity they provide between past and present. Seeing old movies they have seen before can bring back memories. New movies are one way that people can keep in touch with current culture. Many of the movies that can be shown should contain subjects or concepts that may trigger a response for a discussion or make the participants think constructively.

It is the role of the group leader to evaluate what the participants would enjoy viewing. Movies should be carefully selected, not just randomly shown. Movies that are ethnically oriented, showing, for example, people from native American, Jewish, or Irish backgrounds, often cause the residents to think about their own or others' roots and culture. Travelogues are also very popular, including both places that many actually have visited or where many have longed to visit. Check with the libraries in your area for films that may be borrowed or rented. A listing of some loan sources is given in Appendix A.

Lobby Games. There is no limit to the amount of participants in a lobby game, nor is the activity disturbed by the comings and goings of other group members. The following games, all adapted for indoor use, would be useful as activities that can be held in the lobby or gathering place in any facility:

- Shuffleboard
- Safety dart board games
- Ring toss
- Bowling
- Horseshoes

Television game shows make excellent sources of ideas for lobby games. Residents tend to be familiar with the rules of playing such games and enjoy participating in them. Word games are another form of lobby game. Using a large blackboard or some oaktag paper, the residents can suggest a large word from which smaller words may be formed.

Lobby games can be integrated as part of a program of regularly scheduled activities. They are successfully held, for example, before meals. They also can be substituted when a regularly scheduled activity is cancelled. It is possible to utilize the services of volunteers to organize these games. Both participants and observers benefit greatly from this type of activity.

PHYSICAL AILMENTS AND ACTIVITY SUGGESTIONS

This section is an outline of activities that should be either avoided or encouraged, depending on the physical ailments of individuals in a group. We will discuss these in the context of some of the more common ailments.

Arthritis

Arthritis is an inflammation of a joint, usually accompanied by pain. It can result from infection, trauma, or a degenerative joint disease. The following is a list of some rules to follow when planning activities for individuals suffering from arthritis, especially arthritis in the hands.

1. Avoid strong grasping and pinching activities.
2. Press water from cloths or sponges, rather than wringing them.
3. Show participants how to use proximal body parts rather than their fingers. For example, a pocketbook or shopping bag may be slipped on the forearm.
4. Avoid pressure that pushes the participants' knuckles or wrist joints outward.
5. Turn handles or lids toward thumb (inward).
6. Use no craft in which muscles remain in one position for any length of time, such as knitting and crocheting.
7. Stop immediately any activity that produces pain.
8. Try to select an activity so that only noninvolved joints are used

Recent Injuries or Fractures

1. Only light exercise should be given.
2. Active exercise within limits of motion may be used. Graduate the amount of activity, increasing it as the individual improves.

Diabetes

Diabetes is a disease in which the regulation of glucose in the body is disturbed. It can have several symptoms. The following list addresses the activity needs of individuals with diabetes.

1. Avoid activities with sharp instruments. Diabetics are prone to infection, so any cut or abrasion should receive immediate first aid.
2. There is occasional loss of sensation in the fingers of diabetics. Be careful when using heat, for example, when baking or cooking. When participants are sitting at a sink, make sure the drain under the sink is wrapped with tape to prevent burns.
3. In any instance where there is a loss of sensation in the fingers or palms of hands, great care must be taken that the craft selected is not one where friction may produce ulceration or damage to the skin.

Epilepsy

Epilepsy is caused by disturbances in brain function. It is characterized by bodily malfunctions, including convulsions.

1. Do not give epileptic participants sharp tools if seizures are unpredictable.
2. Epileptics who are on medication may be slow in reactions and appear drowsy. Allow for some extra time.

Visual Handicaps

1. The work area should be set up precisely as the participant is to work. The recreation director should draw a map of it, so that every time the person comes to the workshop each tool is in the same place.
2. Before instructing the individual, the recreation director should try the activity personally, blindfolded. If it appears too difficult, break it down into smaller and slower steps.
3. When an individual is introduced to the work area, she should feel the position of each object. The recreation director should tell the individual specifically where each tool is. (Example: "Your pliers are on your right side, three inches from the edge of the bench. The copper wire is 10 inches in front of you in a coil.")
4. For individuals who are temporarily unable to see, or for those recently and suddenly blinded, the sensitivity of hands affects the speed of learning. During this period, feeling must replace sight. Encourage the individual to develop his sense of touch.

5. Make sure the light is adequate for those with visual impairments. People with bifocals or trifocals must have their work placed at the correct distance.

Hearing Disabilities

1. Speak at slightly greater than normal intensity, but do not yell.
2. Speak at a slightly less than normal rate.
3. Speak to the person at a distance of between three and six feet.
4. Never speak directly into a person's ear.
5. If the person does not appear to understand what is being said, rephrase the statement rather than simply repeating the misunderstood words.
6. Do not force the person to listen to you when there is a great deal of background noise.
7. Do not overarticulate. This not only distorts sounds of speech but also the speaker's face, thus making more difficult the receiver's use of visual cues and lip reading.
8. Arrange the room so that no speaker is more than six feet from or only partly visible to any auditorily impaired listener. If possible, try to have a microphone available.

Stroke

Stroke is an injury to the brain that results in an onset of paralysis. It can affect the ability to move major bodily portions. People are affected on the left side as follows:

1. Spatial and visual perception on the left side are damaged. Place the project to be worked on toward the unaffected right side.
2. There are often disturbances in body image that cause a failure to recognize one's own body parts, particularly the affected arms and legs.
3. Often there are disturbances in spatial judgment or relative size and distance of objects. Help the participant to find and work with objects.
4. There also may be disturbances in visual perception, including judgment of vertical and horizontal. Make sure objects are near and easy to reach.

People are affected on the right side in ways similar to the left side, but have some additional problems:

1. They often have difficulty distinguishing between left and right. Avoid the use of directional words as much as possible.
2. Stroke victims generally are:
   a. Poor observers of their environment
   b. Highly suggestible and fluctuate in mental ability
   c. Highly distractable and have a limited attention span

As much as possible, try to get stroke victims to use their affected extremity for performing functional activities. Make sure the person knows what is expected. Never suggest that their lack of attention is due to disinterest.

Chronic Obstructive Pulmonary Disease

Chronic obstructive pulmonary (lung) disease, or COPD, can be due to chronic bronchitis, emphysema, and other similar diseases. Observe the following:

1. A well-ventilated room is essential.
2. When the participant exerts any effort it should be done as she breathes out. Avoid having her lift heavy objects.
3. Avoid using chemicals that may be lung irritants, especially those having strong smells.
4. Avoid stuffings that may be lung irritants.
5. Try to avoid a lot of moving around from one area to another.

Parkinson's Disease

Parkinson's disease is a chronic disorder characterized by tremors, weakness, and rigidity. Individuals with Parkinson's disease suffer from a lack of coordination, loss of facial expression, lowered volume of voice, and a shuffling gait. The person often feels self-conscious and gradually tends to become reclusive, with resulting psychological reactions. Activities for individuals suffering from Parkinson's disease should be encouraged and should consist of

1. Active motion stressing mobility and rapid, rhythmic movements
2. Grasping an object while doing an activity; this has been found to be effective in reducing tremor.

Individuals who work with these people must be aware of the side-effects of anti–Parkinsonian drugs. Observe behaviors of the participants carefully and report changes that might otherwise be missed.

Heart Problems

1. Signs of fatigue that the recreation director should watch for are:
   a. Increased pulse rate
   b. Dyspnea (shortness of breath)
   c. Palpitation
2. Great care must be taken with regard to the participants' posture. See that the individual is comfortable while at work, avoiding eyestrain and jerking movements.

Disturbances in Mental Status

In previous chapters we have seen that old age can be a time of great change. These changes produce stress that can result in feelings of helplessness and hopelessness. It is for this reason that the period of old age is one where there is a great deal of mental illness. Signs of mental illness in the aged may not be indicators of an irreversible problem but rather indicative of loneliness and isolation (Bennett, 1980).

One very efficient way to combat feelings of isolation is through group support (Burnside, 1984). Individuals who share similar concerns, have similar backgrounds, and have had the same experiences tend to give one another the kind of emotional support that is needed to get through the rough times that may develop. This support need not be only at formal group discussions but also can occur at other group activities, such as arts and crafts or even exercise groups. Keeping active and just knowing that there are others around to help, if help is needed, is very important for the maintenance of a healthy mental outlook.

Recreation and socialization groups also assist in establishing a link with reality. This reality is maintained by going to regularly scheduled meetings, including knowing the time of day and day of week that the meetings take place. Taking part in an exhilarating project and seeing it through to its completion are also important aspects.

Being with others in a constructive atmosphere can remove feelings of loneliness and thereby improve mental status.

Illness and Loss

Since activities programs have to be suited to the needs of individuals, in a population where there is a mixture of illnesses, separate activities should be included in the overall group.

Illness in old age, even minor illness, can be a major setback for the individual. In institutional settings where residents may take on the feel of an extended family, illness in one individual can be a setback for the entire group. These setbacks are even more serious when a separation such as hospitalization or death takes place. Older adults, as a result of their age and life experiences, have had to deal with illness and separation in the past. Often they have developed within themselves a means of coping with these problems. It must be clear, however, that, in order for the individual to work through the sorrow of separation, an opportunity should be provided. This can be done only when the staff working with an older adult allows this, which occasionally is difficult for staff, for they have not yet developed their own methods of coping with separation and loss. Staff can learn to deal with their problems at regularly held in-service training sessions. Residents, however, should be given the opportunity to express their feelings during activities. Separation is a fact and therefore should never be concealed.

If a group member has gone to the hospital, for example, it is the staff's responsibility to be aware of that person's condition and to transmit that information when asked for by the other group members. The activities leader should not regard any activity as an inappropriate time to discuss separation. It is easier to deal with loss when the truth is known than when rumor provides the only information.

Memorial services can be held for participants who have died. Gifts of condolence may be sent to the families. These activities represent not just a socially accepted form of remembering others in their time of grief but also help the participants to deal with their own bereavement.

SUMMARY

This chapter described the four categories of activities: (1) discussion groups, (2) physical activities, (3) board games, and (4) other special activities. A discussion followed on how to adapt activities to the special needs of individuals suffering chronic illness. As with other kinds of programs, activity programs for socialization and recreation should be evaluated for their effectiveness. In the next and final chapter, we will look at how to go about conducting a program evaluation.

8

Evaluating Program Effectiveness

We all recognize that the primary goal of providing services to the aged is to respond to the needs of this group of individuals. But once we have begun the programs, how are we to know how effective they are? To respond to this question requires examining or evaluating program effectiveness.

Program evaluation can be defined as the application of research methodology and techniques to the examination and description of issues in real-life settings (Poister, 1978). In the previous chapters, we explored needs assessment and individual evaluation methods and how these techniques were applied in analyzing a variety of programmatic issues. Research on the effectiveness of programs is simply the application of similar principles on a broader scale. Indeed, most funded programs require that ongoing evaluation be performed.

The evaluation process can be used to provide a measure of accountability. Evaluation is not simply a research tool but is also a method of assessing the quality of a program or project. To insure that a program has met its stated objectives and eventually will meet its long-term goals requires measuring data that the program has generated while it has been in operation. The data must then be analyzed. If the program has achieved its objectives then the program is operating well. If not, and if the evaluation process is sufficiently sensitive, weak points in the program's design or implementation procedures may be discovered. If remedied, the program may then achieve its goals.

VALIDITY

Before performing actual evaluation, one must understand what is to be measured and how to apply the correct evaluation tool. This issue is one of validity, which sometimes is defined as truthfulness or accuracy. There is, however, a more technical definition that includes two types of validity, namely, *internal validity* and *external validity* (Campbell & Stanley, 1963).

Internal Validity

Internal validity is defined as the best approximation of knowing that a relationship exists between what is being measured and the results. We say "best approximation" because we can never know for sure if there is a cause–effect relationship between any two objects (Cooke & Campbell, 1979). An example of internal validity is in the measuring of white blood cell counts in an individual with pneumonia. Is there a relationship between the two variables, white blood cell count and pneumonia? We cannot say for sure, but we do know that whenever an individual does have pneumonia their white blood cell count will be elevated. We know that, whenever an individual has an infectious disease, white blood cells increase in number as part of the body's own defenses, to fight off the disease. Our findings then can be considered to be a valid measurement; there is a very close relationship between getting pneumonia and having a higher white blood cell count. It would be wrong, however, to suggest that having a higher white blood cell count is the *cause* of pneumonia.

A more difficult problem arises in social and human service situations. If, for example, we are the director of a senior citizens' center and we believe that, as a result of our programs, older adults in the community are healthier, how can we measure or know that for sure? It may be that our nutritional, educational, and health-screening programs were effective. Or it may be that the local hospital recently had an outreach program that resulted in the change, or local physicians became more active, or the local media urged the aged to take better care of themselves, or healthier older adults have joined our program.

These other sources—the hospital, the doctors, the media, and the clients themselves—are all called *competing factors* or *competing explanations*. To evaluate our program's effectiveness requires us to control for these factors. The better we are able to control the competing explanations, the more confidence we may have in our internal validity. In this particular example we may control the competing explanations by asking the participants if they had any contact with the other sources. If they hadn't and their health status improved, we can feel a little more secure regarding our findings and can say that it would appear that our evaluation has good internal validity.

External Validity

External validity is the degree of generalizability of our findings. If individuals with pneumonia always have elevated white blood cell counts, regardless of their race, social status, or living environment, we can say that an individual with pneumonia will have an elevated white blood count, and the statement will be valid. This, however, may not be true in individuals whose body immune systems do not operate correctly and do not respond to infection. We might, therefore, be forced to re-evaluate our findings to control for cases like this, saying instead that most people who have pneumonia will show a concomitant rise in white blood cell count. Please note, also, that the reverse is not true. If an individual has an elevated white blood cell count, that does not necessarily mean that he has pneumonia. If one were to assume that this were true, that statement would prove not to have good internal validity.

Using our second example, we would be hard pressed to generalize our findings (that health status improved as a result of attendance at a senior citizens' center) to other senior centers, without additional independent proof.

Threats to Validity

In program evaluation, the major concern is with internal validity. Threats to the measurement of internal validity fit into one of three categories:

1. Bias, or systematic error
2. Random error
3. Confound

If there is a *systematic error* in the measurement between variables or items being evaluated, our results will be erroneous. This threat, known as *bias*, may be due to not defining clearly the issue to be measured, and thus to measuring the wrong one. It also can occur as a result of a variety of *testing effects* that change the situation simply by virtue of their being applied. An example might be if we videotaped patients in a clinic and they were aware of the camera. Seeing the camera taking pictures of them might cause the patients to change their normal behavior. They may be more polite or may act more foolish to get attention. This would create a bias in the measurement.

If we use the wrong statistical techniques, or if a random array of factors affect the evaluation, *random error* enters into measurement.

Finally, the worry regarding *confound* is primarily whether or not a causal inference can be supported. Is the construct or issue we say we are measuring the one actually being evaluated? Are we measuring it in its entirety? These are the types of issues that cause questions regarding confounds.

No measurement is without some threat, but often great pains are made to insure the minimalization of these threats.

We have seen in the previous chapters that there exists a variety of tools and methods with which to assess older adults. There are life-satisfaction scales, depression inventories, measures of physical activity level, and a variety of assessment batteries. We also have seen that some of the scales do not measure with a high degree of reliability. This is particularly true of verbatim records or process counseling notes. When we apply scales with low reliability as measuring tools, we are causing error to enter into the measurement. Yet in certain instances we are left with no choice, for better measurement techniques simply may not exist. In cases such as these, it would be wise to use more than one measuring scale. This would provide a degree of *convergent validity* (Campbell & Fiske, 1959). If both measures yield similar findings, then we are more confident of the results. There is no hard-and-fast rule to apply as to what measuring device to use when evaluating which program, but it always is appropriate to use more than one.

THE FIVE EVALUATION QUESTIONS

This section is devoted to the five questions necessary to performing an evaluation. These questions are as follows:

1. The "What" Question. Clearly and operationally define
   a. Long-term goals
   b. Specific program objectives
2. The "Who" Question. Who will be evaluated—staff, program participants, volunteers?
3. The "Where" Question.
   a. What kind of information or data will be needed to perform an accurate evaluation?
   b. Do those data exist?
   c. Where can they be found?
   d. Are these direct data or indirect?
4. The "When" Question.
   a. When did the program begin?

   b. Are there different starting dates for different parts of the program?
5. The "How" Question.
   a. What techniques will be used to analyze the data?
   b. Will the evaluation consist of both formative and summative components?

Basic issues related to these five questions now will be discussed.

The "What" Question

The "what" of the measurement—the exact problem or program to be evaluated—must be clearly understood. It is imperative to define, clearly and operationally, just what it is we are looking at?

In our example from the previous chapter, in which we wanted to involve rural elderly residents in formal recreational and social programs, we may evaluate our success in a variety of ways. When we speak of success, are we referring to the number of people reached, the number of people entering the program, an evaluation of their mental status before entering the program, or several of these factors? None of these issues may be appropriate. To know which ones are the right "what" questions requires clearly understanding the goals and objectives of the program.

If the primary objective is to get as many of the homebound elderly to the senior center, then simply counting those who attend and stating what percent of the rural homebound elderly go to the center is sufficient. If the goal is to have a positive impact on the individual's overall level of well-being, we need a number of measures, possibly including life satisfaction, health status, and mental status, which could begin to provide us with the data necessary to evaluate the program's effectiveness in achieving that goal.

The "Who" Question

The primary "Who" question is: Who are the program participants, and how are they defined? By how they are defined, we mean how they are measured, for example, what their characteristics are and the type of group they make up or belong to.

Other issues often arise during this process, such as, if there is no measurement of participants from the time they started the program until the time of evaluation, how do we know if there is a change? Is there a group of other individuals to whom they may be compared?

Are the others who have been selected for the comparison equivalent to the original group?

If baseline or intake measures do exist, it is important to control for the effects that result from giving the test more than once. These include practice, knowing what the tester wants to see, and other similar confounds. It is also important to determine whether those whom we wish to measure are willing to take part in a research project. Will these individuals be available for follow-up surveys?

These are serious questions, because it has been found that older adults are not particularly interested in being subjects of research studies (Leader & Neuwirth, 1978; Maddox, 1970). Even in instances where the elderly do not have to respond directly to an evaluator, there may be difficulty in gaining permission to see their case files. One possible method for overcoming this difficulty is by carefully explaining the goals of the evaluation procedure and indicating how the respondents may benefit from it.

Elderly program participants are not the only individuals who are disinterested in evaluation or unwilling to take part in it. Staff, too, may be apprehensive about the evaluation process. There may be some fear, usually erroneous, that the assessment will point to specific weaknesses in their own work. This anxiety is often alleviated by having the staff take part in and completely understand the purpose of the evaluation (Weiss, 1975).

The "Where" Question

There are times when evaluation is made part of a program from its inception. This makes the evaluator's task somewhat easier. The goals have been clearly stated and prioritized, and data that reflect progress toward those goals are collected regularly, as part of the project. In these instances, the programs are often designed as research projects and have appropriate controls built in. In cases where evaluation is performed post hoc, that is, after the program is under way or completed, a variety of difficult research questions exist. This type of evaluation is often referred to as *quasi-experimental*, which suggests that it is more difficult to control for competing explanations in such situations.

The first and most pressing problem in a post hoc evaluation is finding out if sufficient data exist with which to perform the evaluation, and, if so, where? Are there attendance records or counseling records? Are there medical charts, or is there a file of requests for service?

Oftentimes records exist and can be located, but these records do not relate directly to the "what" question of the evaluation. At times, a case may be made that, even though the available data are not exactly the same kind of information that is needed to assess the goals of the program, they are similar, and improvement in one area may signal that the program is nearing its goals. One example of this might be in the case where a health clinic program is designed to increase the overall functional status of its older adult participants. As we have seen previously, functional status is a difficult construct to define operationally; therefore, it is difficult to measure. Yet there are some scales that, if used properly, may indicate the overall level of a person's functional status (Salamon, 1982). Using life-satisfaction measures, a measure of physical ability, and progress notes from the individual's case file may all contribute to an understanding of the person's overall functional status.

Another aspect of the "where" question is related even more directly to the goals of the project: Is the project a *global* one, or is it *domain specific?* A *global* question is one of *general* functional assessment, in which a broad number of items related to one overall issue are looked at. A *domain-specific* question is one in which a very clearly delineated item is examined. An example of a domain-specific issue would be how people function in a recreational group.

Sometimes the two types of questions are confused. This can happen in cases where we say, without any justification, that those individuals who attend the recreation group have improved their overall level of functioning. If we are assessing functioning only in the recreation group, we must specify that operationally in our evaluation conclusions. Now it may be that overall functioning is improved as a result of attending the recreation program, but, unless we evaluate that, we cannot draw that conclusion.

The "When" Question

Another important issue to be addressed is when the program actually began. Did the program begin at the outreach stage, or did it start only when the individual entered the actual program? This is an important issue for a variety of reasons. If, from our evaluation, we conclude that the program has successfully achieved its goals, we may find that others wish to copy our project in a different setting. While this is also a question of external validity, in order for the program to be properly transferred to a different location, the details must be specified. If the evaluation indicated that the outreach performed before the program actually started was a contributing factor to the success of the program, then someone wishing to copy the program should know of the importance of that stage of program development.

In terms of service to clients, the "when" question is one in which the *placebo effect* may have to be controlled for and evaluated. The placebo effect occurs when people change or improve simply because they believe in the treatment they are receiving, even though the treatment may have no effect. For example, very isolated elderly may improve in their mental status and show signs of diminishing depression simply as the result of a telephone call, not necessarily because they have joined in a new program. If a telephone call is part of the program and is included in the evaluation study, this effect may be noted as part of the "where" and "what" questions. "Where" asks for information on when the phone calls were made, and "what" asks how the telephone calls contributed to the overall program goals. If such factors are not included in the assessment, we may find that the new program, by itself, is not successful in changing the depression level of its participants.

The "How" Question

Which statistical or evaluative techniques are the appropriate ones to use is the "how" question of evaluation. There are generally two approaches to addressing this question, both of which complement each other.

Summative Component. When an evaluation of a program is based on, for example, the number of telephone calls it receives and the information provided to the caller, the assessment is a purely arithmetic one. This type of assessment is called *summative.* The available information can be summed or combined mathematically.

If the only goal of a program were information and referral, then a summative evaluation of the number of calls and number of appropriate referrals would be sufficient to determine if the goal were achieved. If, on the other hand, the goals were not only to provide information and make a referral, but to act as an advocate to see that the callers received the appropriate service, additional techniques would need to be used. A follow-up survey might be sent to the caller to elicit information for the followup. Inasmuch as the survey is based on rankings, or can be arithmetically combined to yield a sum subject to statistical analysis, the procedure is summative.

Formative Component. If the survey consists of open-ended questions to which the respondents can reply in whatever way they would like, the evaluation takes on a different character. This procedure attempts to categorize the number of times a specific word, feeling, or item is expressed and then to evaluate the factor statistically. This approach may be considered summative; however, it is a difficult procedure and is quite time consuming. Still, it may be no better than simply and concisely reporting the responses in words rather than in statistics. The statistical approach is called a *formative* or *process evaluation*. In this procedure, the overall form of the program is evaluated. Other types of formative evaluations consist of examining case file records, progress notes, and the minutes of staff conferences.

Examples of questionnaires that can be used in program evaluations can be seen in Tables 8–1 and 8–2. Table 8–1 is an example of a follow-up survey for an information-and-referral program. Notice that the questions have clearly specified response choices. These can be easily tabulated to yield response totals. Table 8–2 contains a survey with questions similar to Table 8–1 but the questions in Table 8–2 are open-ended. That is, they allow the respondent to write any response they feel is appropriate.

Table 8–1 Information-and-Referral Follow-up Survey

We are evaluating the I & R program's functioning. You can help us by responding to a few questions. Thank you in advance for taking time out to answer this survey. Please check the appropriate box as to how you feel regarding each question.

1. Was the operator pleasant when you called the I & R program number?
   ☐ Very rude ☐ Unpleasant ☐ Indifferent ☐ Pleasant ☐ Very pleasant
2. Did the phone counselor understand your needs?
   ☐ Did not understand at all ☐ Understood only a little ☐ Understood everything
3. Was the phone counselor able to give you information?
   ☐ Yes ☐ No
4. Was the information you received correct?
   ☐ Yes ☐ No
5. Was the phone counselor helpful in helping you have your needs met?
   ☐ Not at all helpful ☐ Unhelpful ☐ Indifferent ☐ Somewhat helpful ☐ Very helpful.

If you wish to make any comments please use the remaining space.

____
____
____

Table 8–2 Information-and-Referral Follow-up Questionnaire

We are evaluating the I & R program's functioning. You can help us by answering a few questions. Please answer in the spaces provided. Thank you for taking the time out to do so.

1. Did you find the operator pleasant and courteous when you called the I & R program?

2. Were you satisfied with the way the phone counselor spoke to you?

3. Did you find the phone counselor to be helpful?

4. In what way did the phone counselor help you?

5. Was the phone counselor helpful in getting you assistance?

A CASE STUDY

The following is a case study of a program evaluation project. It is based on an actual attempt to evaluate the impact, on the well-being of community-dwelling older adults, of joining a preventive health care program adjacent to a senior citizens' center (Salamon, Charytan, & McQuade, 1982).

The original project was begun as a demonstration program, funded by a private foundation interested in maintaining the quality of life of the elderly who resided in the community. The initial mandate of the program was simply to develop and implement a program whereby a nurse and social worker would provide preventive health care to older adults in offices adjacent to the senior center that they attended.

Immediately prior to the inception of the program, the funding institution's project officer indicated an interest in evaluating the course and outcome of the program. An evaluation component was hastily added to the project. (Evaluations often are hastily prepared, either immediately before a project begins or after it has been operating for a period of time. While this makes the evaluation that much more difficult, it does not make it impossible.)

The Five Evaluation Questions

Let's begin by exploring how the evaluation of the project was performed, using the five essential questions.

What. The "what" question requires us to define clearly and operationally what the evaluation process is designed to evaluate. The goal of the evaluation was to assess the impact of a preventive health care program on the well-being of elderly community residents who attended senior centers. This is not a clearly operationalized evaluation item. It is, furthermore, a long-term goal. Operationally defining this project included establishing some very specific objectives as well as clearly defining what was meant by both *preventive health care* and *well-being*, two somewhat ambiguous components of the goal.

Deciding on clear definitions was considered the most critical first step. Unless we could all agree on these definitions, we could not agree on program objectives. *Preventive health care* ultimately was defined as a specific range of holistic health services to be provided by a nurse, social worker, and consultant medical specialists, according to the specific needs of each program member. In some instances it could mean seeing to it that individuals received the entitlements necessary to have heating fuel for their home in winter, receive food stamps, visit a dentist, or receive physical therapy. Furthermore, specific preventive health interventions were defined according to the three theoretically defined levels of prevention, as detailed in Chapter 2.

The meaning of *well-being* also was defined broadly to include a variety of measures, including scales of life satisfaction; self-reported health; satisfaction with the services provided; and objective measures of health such as days in hospital, visits to health care providers, and outcomes of the visits. An important note is that it was not hypothesized that a change in the number of visits to health care providers would be considered as a measure of well-being. As we discussed previously, the elderly tend to utilize health care services inappropriately; therefore, it was not the actual number of visits that was important, but whether the visits were proper.

Once these definitions had been agreed upon, it was easier to establish some criteria and specify objectives. The first objective was that well-being, as defined, would be measured when each individual registered for the project. A second objective was that all registrants would have a care plan devised, specifying their own areas of need, goals for responding to those needs, and a suggested date for follow-up, either for referral to an outside consultant or for recall by in-house staff.

Who. The "who" question asks us to specify the individuals to be evaluated. As in most instances, evaluations assess not only projects but the individuals who take part in the program. In this program, the who of the evaluation included not only the older adults themselves but the individuals who provided the services. The participants' well-being was evaluated over a period of time using those measures already discussed. The staff also was evaluated. This was done to determine whether or not they had provided the services as specified in the objectives. Did they in fact perform baseline evaluations, determine need, and prepare a plan of care? Was there follow up? These and other questions were asked.

Where. The data for this project were available from patient records, thereby addressing the "where" question. However, there were also other sources of data. For instance, as the project developed, it became clear that some vested interests in the neighboring community had questioned whether the program would conflict with services already being provided by other agencies. This political issue could have had a serious impact on whether people would be encouraged to join the program and whether once they joined, they would continue to receive care from those community providers to which the preventive health care program referred them. This problem was not measurable by clearly specified data, and no objective sources existed. What was done was to make a concerted outreach effort to other providers in the community, explaining the program, indicating its nonthreatening nature, and asking other providers to visit the facility.

As a measure of the impact of this effort, registration rates for membership were compared before the outreach was initiated and afterward. This measure was not at all direct and had several flaws because it did not control for competing explanations such as weather or seasonal variations. Yet it provided some indication of change.

When. The fourth question in evaluation is "when" the program began. For the sake of measuring the well-being component of the preventive health care project, it may be possible to suggest that the project began when the first member registered to participate. From the perspective of evaluating overall impact, the project may have begun when it was in its planning stages. In fact, several issues that occurred prior to the inception of the program had important significance for the evaluation. Among these issues were (1) finding the best location to allow access for older adults, (2) becoming licensed by local departments of health and social welfare, (3) working with the vested interests in the community, and (4) performing outreach to prospective project members. Because the evaluation component was added to the project just prior to the registration of the first member, most of the issues were measured post hoc, or after the fact.

How. The "how" of this project evaluation contains both formative and summative components. The formative aspect, which is a measure of the process itself or how well the project moved toward its goals, included the evaluation of the planning stages, the outreach to vested interests, as well as an ongoing measure of the number of individuals who took part in the services provided. All of this information was fed back to both the administration and the care providers, to indicate areas where more work might be needed.

After two years of operation, a summative evaluation of the project was performed. This resulted in summary data of the entire project, including (1) the total number of people seen; (2) their scores on all the measures of well-being, both at intake and when the evaluation was done; (3) any changes in these measures; (4) the total number of individuals receiving specific forms of care; (5) the number of sick days; (6) the number of days in institutions; and so forth.

Conclusions

Even when evaluations are performed and done well, it is not always easy to specify success or whether any of the goals have been completely achieved. Sometimes what the program workers view as success others do not. For instance, at the preventive health care program, staff believed that they were successful. Indeed, one of the signs of success was that people who had not been to a dentist in five years or more finally had a dental examination. Others felt that one of the program's impacts was to increase the cost of providing health care to program participants, with no significant change in their health. Workers responded that small changes in this age group, even though not statistically significant, were in fact significant for participants' well-being.

While debates of this nature may appear disheartening at first, they should not be misconstrued to mean that evaluations cause more problems than they are worth. Quite the opposite is true. Evaluations help to narrow and specify the precise issues. This results in a much better idea of what took place and how it progressed. For instance, without the evaluation one would never know if the preventive health care program had any impact at all. The evaluation helped narrow the debate to the more manageable question of how much change is to be considered significant.

Politics inevitably will enter evaluation, as they do most everything else; nonetheless, evaluation, even when it is not mandated, is an important component of programming. If you follow the five questions of evaluation, designing a program evaluation will not be difficult.

ADDITIONAL ISSUES

To serve a client and successfully evaluate the service, you need the appropriate information. There are times, though, when the most basic information important to evaluation and care is overlooked, sometimes because everyone assumes it exists but no one has bothered to confirm this. In Chapter 5 we examined some difficulties in obtaining accurate information. Some of these problems related to the best source for confirming questionable information, knowing an older adult client's accurate date of birth, and so forth. This section will explore some additional sources of difficulty.

Often program intake forms do not have a place to note the date of the first interview. When attempting to evaluate whether or not there is seasonal variation in registration, or when attempting to explore the effectiveness of a program according to the participants' age, dates become critical.

A similar difficulty relates to inconsistencies in recording other information. A client's first and last names may become confused if not recorded correctly. Care should be taken with punctuation and with consistent application of rules of recording.

While individuals' names are generally not critical factors in evaluation, others, such as educational level and religion, might very well be. If we were to evaluate the impact of bringing college-level courses to a senior center, based on the educational base of the participants, knowing their level of education would become a critical factor, as it impacts upon their ability to comprehend, absorb, and determine whether this was new information or something previously learned. Furthermore, educational level is highly related to socioeconomic status, among other things, so, if an evaluation of socioeconomic need is to be performed, this information may be important.

Similarly, if one were to evaluate the need for religious services for a group of inpatients, simply knowing whether or not they belonged to one of the major religious denominations or a category called "other" is not sufficient. There must be more detailed information—for example, Reform Jew, or which category of Protestant—in order to determine the services needed.

As these examples indicate, the better and more accurate the information provided, the easier and more accurate the evaluation process. It is necessary to stress the importance of keeping accurate and reliable information, not only, as discussed in previous chapters, to enhance the provision of care, but also to perform an evaluation of the program.

SUMMARY

This chapter introduced the reader to some of the issues in assessment of programs and discussed basic evaluation techniques. We explored the issue of validity in measurement and the five questions an evaluator should answer. A case study was provided to illustrate these points.

This discussion is by no means exhaustive, but it does stress the importance of clearly defining a program's goals and objectives. It indicates that if the program is well planned and developed an evaluation will be easier to perform. This does not mean that the evaluation process will always indicate that the program is doing what it initially set out to do. If an evaluation is done correctly, however, it can indicate the strengths and the weak points of a program and suggest means of overcoming any shortcomings.

Appendix A

Film Loan Services

The following is a list of some of the organizations that provide films for little or no cost.

Aetna Life & Casualty
Film Library
151 Farmington Avenue
Hartford, CT 06115

American Cancer Society
219 East 42nd Street
New York, NY 10017

American Heart Association
44 East 23rd Street
New York, NY 10010

American Institute of Architects
Film Librarian
1735 New York Avenue, N.W.
Washington, DC 20006

American National Red Cross
150 Amsterdam Avenue
New York, NY 10023

Arkansas Department of Parks & Tourism
149 State Capitol Building
Little Rock, AK 72201

Armstrong Cork Company
Consumer Services
Liberty & Charlotte Streets
Lancaster, PA 17604

Association-Sterling Films
866 Third Avenue
New York, NY 10021

Bay State Film Productions, Inc.
Box 129
Springfield, MA 01101

Belgian Embassy
Film Library
3330 Garfield Street, N.W.
Washington, DC 20008

Brooklyn Union Gas
P.R. & Advertising Dept.
195 Montague Street
Brooklyn, NY 11201

Bureau of Mines
U.S. Dept. of the Interior
Motion Pictures
4800 Forbes Avenue
Pittsburgh, PA 15213

Bureau of Reclamation
Film Management Center
P.O. Box 25007
Denver Federal Center
Denver, CO 80225

Campbell Films
Film Library
Saxtons River, VT 05154

Caterpillar Tractor Co.
Caterpillar Film Library
1687 Elmhurst Road
Elk Grove Village, IL 60007

Charard Motion Pictures, Inc.
2110 East 24th Street
Brooklyn, NY 11229

Chevron Chemical Company
ORTHO Division
200 Bush Street
San Francisco, CA 94104

Chinese Information Service
3440 Wilshire Boulevard
Los Angeles, CA 90010

Coca-Cola Bottling Co.
Attn: Public Relations Director
74-12 88th Street
Glendale, NY 11227

Consulate General of Finland
540 Madison Avenue
New York, NY 10022

Consulate General of Ireland
580 Fifth Avenue
New York, NY 10036

Consulate General of Japan
c/o Association-Sterling Films
866 Third Avenue
New York, NY 10022

Dawn Film Service
1611 The Midway
Glendale, CA 91208

Department of State
c/o National Audiovisual Center
Distribution Branch
Washington, DC 20409

Department of the Air Force
Air Force Central Audiovisual Library
Norton Air Force Base, CA 92409

Department of the Army
First United States Army
Audio-Visual Support Center
Fort George G. Meade, MD 20755

Department of the Navy
Education & Training Support Center
Film Library
Federal Office Building, 5th Floor
3rd Avenue and 29th Street
Brooklyn, NY 11232

Du Pont De Nemours & Co., Inc.
Motion Picture Section
1007 Market Street
Wilmington, DE 19898

Eastern Air Lines, Inc.
Film Library
International Airport Branch
Miami, FL 33148

Eastman Kodak Co.
Audio-Visual Library
343 State Street
Rochester, NY 14650

Embassy of Argentina
Cultural Office
1600 New Hampshire Ave., N.W.
Washington, DC 20009

Embassy of Finland
1900 24th Street, N.W.
Washington, DC 20008

Embassy of Malaysia
Information & Cultural Attaché
2401 Massachusetts Ave., N.W.
Washington, DC 20008

Embassy of Poland
Press Office
Polish Embassy
2640 Sixteenth Street, N.W.
Washington, DC 20009

Embassy of the State of Kuwait
Film Library
2940 Tilden Street, N.W.
Washington, DC 20008

Exxon Corporation
Public Affairs Dept.
1251 Avenue of the Americas
New York, NY 10020

Farm Film Foundation
1425 H Street, N.W.
Washington, DC 20005

Florida Department of Commerce
Film Library
Collins Building
107 W. Gaines Street
Tallahassee, FL 32304

General Mills, Inc.
9200 Film Center
P.O. Box 1113
Minneapolis, MN 55440

General Motors Corp.
Film Library
General Motors Building
Detroit, MI 48202

Goodyear Tire & Rubber Co.
Film Library
1144 East Market Street
Akron, OH 44316

Greenfield Village & Henry Ford Museum
Audio Visual Services
Department of Education
Dearborn, MI 48121

Grumbacher Film Library
267 West 25th Street
New York, NY 10001

Heinz U.S.A.
Film Department
P.O. Box 57
Pittsburgh, PA 15230

Ideal Pictures Film Library
4431 West North Avenue
Milwaukee, WI 53208

Information Service of India
Film Section
3 East 64th Street
New York, NY 10021

International Business Machines
Modern Talking Picture Service
1212 Avenue of the Americas
New York, NY 10036

Italian Cultural Institute
Audio Visual Department
686 Park Avenue
New York, NY 10021

Japan Air Lines
c/o Association-Sterling Films
600 Grand Avenue
Ridgefield, NJ 07657

Japan National Tourist Organization
45 Rockefeller Plaza
New York, NY 10020

Jewish Chautauqua Society
Film Librarian
838 Fifth Avenue
New York, NY 10021

Johnson Outboards
Solana Studios
4365 N. 27th Street
Milwaukee, WI 53216

Kentucky Department of Public Information
Film Library
Capitol Annex Building
Frankfort, KY 40601

Klein Company
Distribution Director
6301 Carmel Road
Charlotte, NC 28211

Lilly & Company
Audio Visual Film Library
P.O. Box 618
Indianapolis, IN 46206

Lockheed-Georgia Co.
Film Library
Zone 30, B-2 Building
Marietta, GA 30063

McDonnell Douglas Corp.
Film & TV Communications
3000 Ocean Park Boulevard
Santa Monica, CA 90406

McDonnell Douglas Corp.
Film Library
Department 091
P.O. Box 516
St. Louis, MO 63166

Maine Department of Agriculture
Motion Picture Services
State Office Building
Augusta, ME 04330

Marathon Oil Company
Film Library
539 South Main Street
Findlay, OH 45840

Master Chemical Corp.
501 West Boundary
Perrysburg, Ohio 43551

Mercedes-Benz
Film Library
Dept. of Creativision
295 West 4th Street
New York, NY 10014

Miller Brewing Company
Film Library
4000 West State Street
Milwaukee, WI 53208

Missouri Tourism Commission
Film Librarian
308 East High Street
P.O. Box 1055
Jefferson City, MO 65101

Modern Talking Picture Service
315 Springfield Avenue
Summit, NJ 07901

Motion Picture Services
P.O. Box 252
Livingston, NJ 07039

NASA Film Library
National Audiovisual Center
Washington, DC 20409

National Gallery of Art
Extension Service
Washington, DC 20565

National Oceanic and Atmospheric
Administration
U.S. Dept. of Commerce
Motion Picture Service
12231 Wilkens Avenue
Rockville, MD 20852

National Society for the Prevention of
Blindness, Inc.
Public Information Department
79 Madison Avenue
New York, NY 10016

New Zealand Films
c/o Association-Sterling Films
600 Grand Avenue
Ridgefield, NJ 07657

Permanent Mission of Malaysia to the
United Nations
666 Third Avenue, 30th Floor
New York, NY 10017

Picadilly Films International
Box 16255, Lapham Station
San Antonio, TX 78246

Planters Peanuts
Arthur Mokin Productions
17 West 60th Street
New York, NY 10023

Portuguese National Tourist and
Information Service
570 Fifth Avenue
New York, NY 10036

Public Service Audience Planners
545 Fifth Avenue
New York, NY 10017

Quebec Government House
The Film Officer
Rockefeller Plaza
17 West 50th Street
New York, NY 10020

Reynolds Metals Company
Motion Picture Services
P.O. Box 27003
Richmond, VA 23261

Rhode Island Developmental Council
Rhode Island Library Film Cooperative
c/o Warwick Public Library
600 Sandy Lane
Warwick, RI

RHR Film Media, Inc.
48 West 48th Street
New York, NY 10036

Royal Danish Consulate General
Danish Information Office
280 Park Avenue
New York, NY 10017

Santa Fe Film Library
316 Railway Exchange
Chicago, IL 60604

Sikorsky Aircraft
Public Relations Department
Stratford, CT 06602

Solana Studios
Film Distribution Center
4365 North 27th Street
Milwaukee, WI 53216

STP Corporation
Film Librarian
1400 W. Commercial Blvd.
Fort Lauderdale, FL 33310

Swiss National Tourist Office
c/o Tribune Films, Inc.
38 West 32nd Street
New York, NY 10001

Telefilm Ltd.
P.O. Box 709
Homosassa Springs, FL 32647

Tennessee Valley Authority
Film Services
Knoxville, TN 37902

Texaco, Inc.
1040 Kings Highway North
Cherry Hill, NJ 08002

Thiokol Corporation
Film Library
P.O. Box 27
Bristol, PA 19007

Tourist Organization of Thailand
20 East 82nd Street
New York, NY 10028

Travelers Film Library
Modern Talking Picture Service
2323 New Hyde Park Road
New Hyde Park, NY 11040

Tribune Films, Inc.
38 West 32nd Street
New York, NY 10001

Turkish Tourism & Information
Service
500 Fifth Avenue
New York, NY 10036

United Jewish Appeal
Public Relations: Films
1290 Sixth Avenue
New York, NY 10019

United States Atomic Energy
Commission
Film Library
P.O. Box 62
Oak Ridge, TN 37830

United States Coast Guard
Third Coast Guard District
Commander
Governors Island
New York, NY 10004

United States Postal Service
Main Post Office
New York, NY 10098

United States Steel Corporation
71 Broadway
New York, NY 10006

West Glen Films
565 Fifth Avenue
New York, NY 10017

Westinghouse Electric Corp.
Visual Communications Dept.
Westinghouse Building
Gateway Center
Pittsburgh, PA 15222

West Virginia Department of
Commerce
Travel Development Division
State Office Building #6
1900 Washington Street, East
Charleston, WV 25305

Appendix B

Health-education Materials

The following is a list of some of the organizations that provide health-education materials at little or no cost.

Alcoholism

Aetna Life & Casualty
151 Farmington Avenue
Hartford, CT 06115

Association for the Advancement of Health Education
1201 Sixteenth Street, N.W.
Washington, DC 20036

Kemper Insurance
Advertising & Public Relations Dept.
110 Tenth Avenue
Fulton, IL 61252

National Council on Alcoholism
2 Park Avenue
New York, NY 10016

National Institute on Alcohol Abuse and Alcoholism
National Institute of Mental Health
5600 Fishers Lane
Rockville, MD 20852

Allergies

Allergy Foundation of America
801 Second Avenue
New York, NY 10017

National Institute of Allergy & Infectious Diseases
Office of Information
Bethesda, MD 20014

Arthritis and Rheumatism

The Arthritis Foundation
GPO Box 2525
New York, NY 10036

Cancer

American Cancer Society, Inc.
Vice President for Public Education
219 East 42nd Street
New York, NY 10017

Cystic Fibrosis

National Cystic Fibrosis Research Foundation
60 East 42nd Street
New York, NY 10017

Diabetes

American Diabetes Association
1 West 48th Street
New York, NY 10020

Drug Dependence and Abuse

Connecticut General Life Insurance Company
Advertising & Public Relations–319
Hartford, CT 06115

Kemper Insurance
Advertising & Public Relations Department
110 Tenth Avenue
Fulton, IL 61252

National Institute of Drug Abuse/DHEW
11400 Rockville Pike
Rockville, MD 20852

Pharmaceutical Manufacturers Association
Public Relations Division
1155 Fifteenth Street, N.W.
Washington, DC 20005

Epilepsy

Epilepsy Foundation of America
1828 L Street, N.W., Suite 406
Washington, DC 20036

Genetic Disease

National Genetics Foundation
250 West 57th Street
New York, NY 10019

Heart Disease

American Heart Association
Inquiries Section
44 East 23rd Street
New York, NY 10010

Kidney Disease

National Kidney Foundation
116 East 27th Street
New York, NY 10010

Leukemia

Leukemia Society of America
211 East 43rd Street
New York, NY 10017

Multiple Sclerosis

National Multiple Sclerosis Society
Public Relations Dept.
257 Park Avenue South
New York, NY 10010

Muscular Dystrophy

Muscular Dystrophy Associations of America, Inc.
Public Information Department
810 Seventh Avenue
New York, NY 10019

Obesity

Connecticut General Life Insurance Company
Advertising & Public Relations–319
Hartford, CT 06115

Liberty Mutual Insurance Co.
Public Relations Dept.
175 Berkeley Street
Boston, MA 02117

Metropolitan Life Insurance Co.
Health & Welfare Division
1 Madison Avenue
New York, NY 10010

Parkinson's Disease

National Parkinson Foundation, Inc.
(Supports the National Parkinson Institute for Treatment & Rehabilitation. Also supports the Bob Hope Parkinson Research Institute.)
1501 N.W. Ninth Avenue
Miami, FL 33136

Respiratory Diseases

American Lung Association
1740 Broadway
New York, NY 10019

Smoking and Health

American Heart Association
Inquiries Section
44 East 23rd Street
New York, NY 10010

American Lung Association
1740 Broadway
New York, NY 10019

National Clearinghouse for Smoking and Health
U.S. Public Health Service
5600 Fishers Lane
Rockville, MD 20852

Tuberculosis

American Lung Association
1740 Broadway
New York, NY 10019

Venereal Disease

American Social Health Association
1740 Broadway
New York, NY 10019

Connecticut General Life Insurance Company
Advertising and Public Relations–319
Hartford, CT 06115

References

Abramson, R., Kahn, B. H., & Rosenbaum, C. (1981). Managing hopelessness in chronic care. *Geriatrics*, 36, 162–164

Allan, C., & Brotman, H. (1981). *Chartbook on aging in America*. Washington, DC: The 1981 White House Conference on Aging.

American Psychiatric Association. (1980). *Diagnostic and Statistical Manual of Mental Disorders* (3rd. ed.). Washington, DC: Author.

Atchley, R. C. (1972). *The social forces in later life*. Belmont, CA: Wadsworth.

Auerbach, A. (1972). The elderly in rural areas: Differences in urban areas and implications for practice. In L. Ginsberg (Ed.), *Social work in rural communities* (pp. 93–121). New York: Council on Social Work Education.

Baddeley, A. (1984). Memory theory and memory therapy. In B. A. Wilson & N. Moffat (Eds.), *Clinical management of memory problems* (pp. 5–27). London: Aspen.

Baldwin, L. F., & Loewinsohn, R. J. (1979). *Widowed Persons Service organization manual*. Washington, D.C.: National Retired Teachers Association/American Association of Retired Persons.

Ballot, R., Clark, J., Fersh, I., Komanoff, H., & Patton, T. (1979). *Teaching about aging*. Long Beach, NY: Long Beach City School District.

Barnes, E. K., & Shore, H. H. (1977). *Holiday programming for long-term care facilities*. Denton, TX: North Texas State University.

Bennett, R. (1976). Attitudes of the young toward the old: A review of research. *Personnel and Guidance Journal*, 55, 136–139.

Bennett, R. (1980). *Aging, isolation and resocialization*. New York: Van Nostrand Reinhold

Berezin, M. A. (1972). Psychodynamic considerations of aging and the aged. *American Journal of Psychiatry*, 128, 220–228.

Berger, M. M., & Berger, L. F. (1971). An innovative program for a private psychogeriatric day center. *Journal of the American Geriatrics Society*, 19, 210–219.

Bloom, B. S., Hastings, J. T., & Madavs, G. F. (1971). *Handbook on formative and summative evaluation of student learning*. New York: McGraw-Hill.

Borup, J. H. (1982). The effects of varying degrees of interinstitutional environmental change on long-term care patients. *Gerontologist*, 22, 409–417.

Botwinick, J., West, J. R., & Storandt, M. (1978) Predicting death from behavior test performance. *Journal of Gerontology*, 33, 755–762.
Bradford, Healthfield Newsletter, (1979, November/December), 2, 1.
Brehm, H. P. (1980). Organization and financing of health care for the aged: Future implications. In S. G. Haynes & M. Feinleib (Eds.), *Second conference on the epidemiology of aging* (pp. 329–348). Bethesda, MD: National Institute of Health.
Breslau, L. D., & Haug, M. R. (Eds.). (1983). *Depression and aging: Causes, care and consequences*. New York: Springer.
Brickfield, C. (1979). *Educating the elderly. The Jewish Journal*, 31, 19–25.
Brink, T. L. (1979). *Geriatric Psychotherapy*. New York: Human Sciences Press.
Brink, T. L. (1980). The myth of the senility myth. *Journal of the National Medical Association*, 72, 1042–1043.
Brody, E. (1978). The aging of the family. *The Annals*, 438, 13–27.
Brody, E., Davis, L. J., Fulcomer, M., & Johnson, P. (1979, November). *Three generations of women: Comparisons of attitudes and preferences for service providers*. Paper presented at the 32nd Annual Meeting of the Gerontological Society of America, Washington, D.C.
Brooks, N., & Lincoln, N. (1984). Assessment for rehabilitation. In B. A. Wilson & N. Moffat (Eds.), *Clinical management of memory problems* (pp. 28–45). London: Aspen.
Brotman, H. B. (1977). Voter participation in November 1976. *Gerontologist*, 17, 157–159.
Buckingham, R. W. (1979). Primary care of the terminally ill. *Geriatrics*, 34, 73–75.
Burnside, I. M. (1984). *Working with the elderly: Group process and techniques* (2nd ed.). Monterey, CA: Wadsworth Health Sciences Press.
Butler, R. N. (1963). The life review: An interpretation of reminiscence in the aged. *Psychiatry*, 26, 65–76.
Butler, R. N. (1975). *Why survive? Being old in America*. New York: Harper & Row.
Butler, R. N., & Lewis, M. (1976). *Sex after sixty*. New York: Harper & Row.
Butler, R. N., & Lewis, M. (1982). *Aging and mental health* (3rd ed.). St. Louis: C. V. Mosby.
Campbell, D. T., & Fiske, D. W. (1959). Convergent and discriminant validation by the multitrait–multimethod matrix. *Psychological Bulletin*, 56, 81–105.
Campbell, D. T., & Stanley, J. C. (1963). *Experimental and quasi-experimental designs for research*. Chicago: Rand-McNally.
Cantor, M. H. (1981). The extent and intensity of the informal support system among New York's inner city elderly—Is ethnicity a factor? In *Strengthening informal supports for the aging: Theory, practice and policy implications*. New York: Community Service Society of New York.
Caplow-Lindner, E., Harpaz, L., & Samberg, S. (1979). *Therapeutic dance and movement: Expressive activities for older adults*. New York: Human Sciences Press.
Carey, R. G. (1979–1980). Weathering widowhood: Problems and adjustments of the widow during the first year. *Omega*, 10, 163–174.
Carp, F. (1977). Housing and living environments of older people. In R. Binstock & E. Shanas (Eds.), *Handbook of aging in the social sciences* (pp. 219–231). New York: Van Nostrand Reinhold.
Clayton, P. J. (1979). The sequelae and non-sequelae of conjugal bereavement. *American Journal of Psychiatry*, 136, 1530–1534.

Cobb, S., & Kasi, S. V. (1977). *Termination: The consequences of job loss*. Cincinnati, OH: U.S. Department of Health Education and Welfare.

Collins, J. A. (1982). Medicare and Medicaid: Cuts and concerns. *Geriatrics, 37*, 33–38.

Conte, V. A., & Salamon, M. J. (1981, September). *Promoting intergenerational understanding: The counselor's and teacher's role in helping children understand older adults*. Paper presented at the 16th Annual Convention of the New York State Professional Guidance Association, Lake Placid, New York.

Cooke, T. D., & Campbell, D. T. (1979). *Quasi-experimentation: Design and analysis issues for field settings*. Chicago: Rand-McNally.

Coppen, A. (1976). The biochemistry of affective disorders. *British Journal of Psychiatry, 113*, 1237–1264.

Costa, P. T. (1984). *Abuse of the elderly*. Lexington, MA: Lexington Books.

Costa, P. T., & McCrae, R. R. (1980). Still stable after all these years: Personality as a key to some issues in adulthood and old age. In P. B. Baltes & O. G. Brim (Eds.), *Life span development and behavior* (vol. 3). New York: Academic Press.

Covey, H. C. (1982). A reconceptualization of continuity theory: Some preliminary thoughts. *Gerontologist, 21*, 628–633.

Cowens, E. L. (1982). Help is where you find it: Four informal helping groups. *American Psychologist, 37*, 384–395.

Croake, J. W., & Glover, K. E. (1977). Understanding old age: The Adlerian perspective. *Geriatrics*, 32, 93–104.

Cumming, E. M., & Henry, W. (1961). *Growing old*. New York: Basic Books.

Cutler, N. R., Duara, R., Creasey, H., Grady, C. L., Haxby, J. V., Schapiro, M. B., & Rapoport, S. I. (1984). Brain imaging: Aging and dementia. *Annals of Internal Medicine, 101*, 355–369.

Daum, M. (1982). Preference for age-homogeneous versus age-heterogeneous social interaction. *Journal of Gerontological Social Work, 4*, 41–55.

Donahue, W., Thompson, M., & Curren, D. (Eds.). (1977). *Congregate housing for older people*. Washington, DC: U.S. Department of Health Education and Welfare.

Ducovney, A. (1969). *The billion dollar swindle: Frauds against the elderly*. New York: Fleet Press.

Ebersole, P. (1976). Reminiscing. *American Journal of Nursing, 76*, 48–52.

Edwards, J., & Klemmack, L. (1973). Correlates of life satisfaction: A reexamination. *Journal of Gerontology*, 28, 497–502.

Eichorn, D. H., Clausen, J. A., Haan, N., Honzik, M. P., & Mussen, P. H. (Eds.), (1981), *Present and past in middle life*. New York, Academic Press.

Eisdorfer, C., & Lawton, M. P. (1973). *The psychology of adult development and aging*. Washington, DC: American Psychological Association.

Engel, G. L. (1971). Sudden and rapid death during psychological stress. *Annals of Internal Medicine*, 74, 683–701.

Erikson, E. H. (1950). *Childhood and Society*. New York, W. W. Norton & Co.

Evans, R. L., & Jaureguy, B. M. (1982). Phone therapy outreach for blind elderly. *Gerontologist*, 22, 32–35.

Federal Council on the Aging. (1981). *The need for long-term care: Information and issues*. Washington, DC: Department of Health and Human Services.

Fengler, A. P., & Goodrich, N. (1979). Wives of elderly disabled men: The hidden patients. *Gerontologist, 19*, 175–183.

Ferguson, R. N. (1976). Hear! Hear! *The Monthly Bulletin of the New York State Office for the Aging*, 9, 10–11.
Frenkel-Brunswik, E. (1968). Adjustments and reorientation in the course of the life span. In B. Neugarten (Ed.), *Middle age and aging*. Chicago: The University of Chicago Press.
Friedman, E. A., & Havighurst, R. J. (1954). *The meaning of work and retirement*. Chicago: University of Chicago Press.
Friedman, M., & Rosenman, R. F. (1974). *Type A behavior and your heart*. New York: Knopf.
Fries, J. F. (1983). The compression of morbidity. *Milbank Memorial Fund Quarterly*, *61*, 397–419.
Furukawa, C., & Shoemaker, D. (1982). *Community health services for the aged: Promotion and maintenance*. Rockville, MD: Aspen.
Gaarder, L. R., & Cohen, S. (1982). *Patient activated care for rural elderly*. Boise, ID: Mountain States Health Corporation.
Gaitz, C. M., McCaslin, R., & Calvert, W. R. (1977). Information and referral: Components of comprehensive care. In C. Eisdorfer & R. O. Friedel, (Eds.), *Cognitive and emotional disturbances in the elderly: Clinical issues* (pp. 70–93). Chicago: Medical Year Book Publishing.
The Gallup Report (1982, June–July). *Religion in America, 1982*. Report nos. 201–202.
Gatz, M., Smyer, M. A., & Lawton, M. P. (1980). The mental health system and the older adult: In L. W. Poon (Ed.), *Aging in the 1980's: Psychological issues* (pp. 5–18) Washington, DC: American Psychological Association.
German, P. S. (1978). The elderly: A target group highly accessible to health education. *International Journal of Health Education*, *21*, 267–272.
Glenn, N. E., & Grimes, M. (1968). Aging, voting and political interest. *American Sociological Review*, 33, 572–573.
Goleman, D. (1982). Coping with death on a long distance line. *Psychology Today*, *16*, 42–48.
Gore, S. (1978). The effect of social support in moderating the health consequences of unemployment. *Journal of Health and Social Behavior*, *19*, 157–165.
Gould, E., & Gould, L. (1971). *Crafts for the elderly*. Springfield, IL.: Charles C. Thomas.
Gray, D. (1983). A job club for older job seekers: An experimental evaluation. *Journal of Gerontology*, 38, 363–368.
Granick, S., & Patterson, R. D. (1971). *Human aging II: An eleven year follow up biomedical and behavioral study*. Rockville, MD: U.S. Public Health Service.
Green, S. K. (1981). Attitudes and perceptions about the elderly: Current and future perspectives. *Aging and Human Development*, *13*, 95–115.
Gurlin, G., Veroff, J., & Feld, S. (1960). *Americans view their mental health*. New York: Basic Books.
Haan, N. (1977). *Coping and defending*. New York: Academic Press.
Halperin, J. (1981). Rewards of home visiting. *Perspectives on Aging*, *10*, 26–27.
Hanan, Z. I. (1978). Geriatric medications: How the aged are hurt by drugs meant to help. *RN*, *11*, 29–32.
Harbert, A. S., & Ginsberg, L. H. (1979). *Human services for older adults: Concepts and skills*. Belmont, CA: Wadsworth.
Hare, P. H. (1982). The empty nest as a golden egg. *Perspective on Aging*, *11*, 21–23.

Harper, D. C. (1984). Application of Orem's theoretical constructs to self-care medication behaviors in the elderly. *Advances in Nursing Science*, 29–46.
Harris, D. K., & Cole, W. E. (1980). *Sociology of aging*. Boston, MA: Houghton Mifflin.
Hastings, L. (1981). *Complete handbook of activities and recreational programs for nursing homes*. Englewood Cliffs, NJ: Prentice-Hall.
Hays, J. A. (1984) Aging and family resources: Availability and proximity of kin. *Gerontologist*, *24*, 149–153.
Hendin, D. (1973). *Death as a fact of life*. New York: Norton.
Hickey, T. (1980). *Health and aging*. Monterey, CA: Brooks/Cole.
Holzberg, L. (1982). Ethnicity and aging: Anthropological perspectives on more than just the minority elderly. *Gerontologist*, *22*, 249–257.
Horn, P. (1975). Smoothing the road to retirement. *Psychology Today*, *9*, 52.
Howells, J. G. (Ed.). (1975). *Modern perspectives in the psychology of old age*. New York: Brunner/Mazel.
Institute of Public Administration. (1975). *Improving transportation services of older americans*. Washington, DC: U.S. Government Printing Office.
Jacobs, B. (Ed.). (1980). *Senior centers and the at-risk older person*. Washington, DC: National Council on Aging
Jacobs, B., Lindsley, P., & Fell, M. (1976). *A guide to intergenerational programming*. Washington, DC: National Institute of Senior Centers.
Jantz, R. K., & Seefeldt, C. (1977). A child's view of the elderly. *Psychology Today*, *10*, 8.
Jarner, R. V., & Verwoerdt, A. (1975). Training of psychogeriatricians. In J. G. Howells (Ed.), *Modern perspectives in the psychiatry of old age* (570–583) New York: Brunner/Mazel.
Johnson, C. L., & Catalano, D. J. (1981). Childless elderly and their family supports. *Gerontologist*, *21*, 610–618.
Jones, R. (1977). *The other generation: The new power of older people*. Englewood Cliffs, NJ: Science Press.
Kahana, E. (1975). Matching environments to the needs of the aged: A conceptual scheme. In J. Gubrium (Ed.), *Late life: Recent developments in the sociology of aging*. Springfield, IL: Charles C Thomas.
Kalish, R. (1975). *Late adulthood: Perspectives on human development*. Monterey, CA: Brooks/Cole.
Kalish, R. (1978). A little myth is a dangerous thing: Research in the service of the dying. In C. Gurfield (Ed.), *Psychosocial care of the dying* (pp. 434–487). New York: McGraw-Hill.
Kane, R. A., & Kane, R. L. (1981). *Assessing the elderly: A practical guide to measurement*. Lexington, MA: Lexington Books.
Kane, R. L., Jorgenson, L. A., Titeberg, B., & Kawahora, J. (1976). Is good nursing home care feasible? *Journal of the American Medical Association*, *235*, 516–519.
Kane, R. L., & Kane, R. A. (1980). Alternatives to institutional care of the elderly: Beyond the dichotomy. *Gerontologist*, *20*, 249–259.
Kartman, L. L. (1979). Therapeutic group activities in nursing homes. *Health and Social Work*, *4*, 135–144.
Kasl, S. V., & Bereman, L. F. (1981). Some psychosocial influences on the health status of the elderly: The perspective of social epidemiology. In G. March (Ed.), *Aging: Biology and behavior* (pp. 345–385). New York: Academic Press.

Kay, D. W. K., & Bergman, K. (1980). Epidemiology of mental disorders among the aged in the community. In J. E. Birren & R. B. Sloane (Eds.), *Handbook of mental health and aging*. Englewood Cliffs, NJ: Prentice-Hall.

Kay, J. G. (1977). *Crafts for the very disabled and handicapped of all ages*. Springfield, IL: Charles C Thomas.

Kernberg, O. F. (1977). Normal psychology of the aging process revisited II. *Journal of Geriatric Psychiatry, 10*, 27–45.

Kogan, L. S. (1957). The short-term case in a family agency. *Social Casework, 38*, 296–302.

Kopf, R., Salamon, M. J., & Charytan, P. (1982). The preventive health history form: A questionnaire for use with older patient populations. *Journal of Gerontological Nursing, 8*, 519–523.

Kos, B. A. (1976). Annual report of the nursing center for family health services. Robert Wood Johnson Foundation (mimeo).

Kovar, M. G. (1980). Morbidity and health care utilization. In D. G. Haynes & M. Feinleib (Eds.), *Second conference on the epidemiology of aging*. Bethesda, MD: National Institute of Health.

Krauss, A. A., & Lillienfeld, A. M. (1959). Some epidemiological aspects of the high mortality rate in the young widowed group. *Journal of Chronic Diseases, 10*.

Kübler-Ross, E. (1979). *On death and dying*, New York: MacMillan Publishing Co.

Kübler-Ross, E. (1979). *Questions and answers on death and dying*. New York: MacMillan Publishing Co.

Kübler-Ross, E. (1975). *Death—The final stage of growth*. Englewood Cliffs, NJ: Prentice Hall.

Kurlychek, R. T. (1983). Use of a digital alarm chronograph as a memory aid in early dementia. *Clinical Gerontologist, 1*, 93–94.

LaCherie, N., Ryan, R., & Barocas, C. (1981). *Problems of the elderly: A needs assessment workbook*. Bethesda, MD: Administration on Aging.

Lareau, L. S., & Heumann, L. F. (1982). The inadequacy of needs assessment of the elderly. *Gerontologist, 22*, 324–339.

Larson, R. (1978). Thirty years of research on the subjective well-being of older Americans. *Journal of Gerontology, 33*, 119–125.

Lashof, J. C. (1977). Do benefits exceed costs of alternatives to institutional care? *Geriatrics, 32*, 33–36.

Lawton, M. P., & Nahemow, L. (1973). Ecology and the aging process. In C. Eisdorfer & M. P. Lawton (Eds.), *The psychology of adult development and aging* (pp. 619–674). Washington, DC: American Psychological Association.

Leader, M. A., & Neuwirth, E. (1978). Clinical research and the noninstitutional elderly: A model for subject recruitment. *Journal of the American Geriatrics Society, 26*, 27–30.

Leinbach, R. M. (1982). Alternatives to the face-to-face interview for collecting gerontological needs assessment data. *Gerontologist, 22*, 78–82.

Lieberman, M. A. (1965). Psychological correlates of impending death: Some preliminary observations. *Journal of Gerontology, 1*, 20–25.

Linn, B. S., & Linn, M. W. (1980). Objective self-assessed health in the old and very old. *Social Science and Medicine, 14*, 311–314.

Lowenthal, M. F. (1965). Antecedents of isolation and mental illness in old age. *Archives of General Psychiatry, 12*, 245–254.

Macheath, J. A. (1984). *Activity, health and fitness in old age*. New York: St. Martin's Press.

Maddison, D., & Viola, A. (1968). The health of widows in the year following bereavement. *Journal of Psychosomatic Research, 12,* 297–310.

Maddox, G. (1970). Selected methodological issues in normal aging. In E. Palmore (Ed.), *The Duke longitudinal study.* Chapel Hill, NC: Duke University Press.

Markides, K. S., & Martin, H. W. (1979). A causal model of life satisfaction among the elderly. *Journal of Gerontology, 34,* 86–93.

Matthews, S. H. (1982). Participation of the elderly in a transportation system. *Gerontologist,* 22, 26–31.

McCaslin, R. (1981). Next steps in information and referral for the elderly. *Gerontologist, 21,* 184–193.

McClanahan, L. E., & Risley, T. R. (1975). Design of living environments for nursing home residents: Increasing participation in recreational activities. *Journal of Applied Behavioral Analysis, 8,* 261–268.

McCormack, D., & Whitehead, A. (1981). The effect of providing recreational activities on the engagement level of long-stay geriatric patients. *Age and Aging, 10,* 287–291.

McKhann, G., Drachman, D., Folstein, M., Katzman, R., Price, D., & Stadlan, E. M. (1984). Clinical diagnosis of Alzheimer's disease: Report of the NINCDS-ADRDA Work Group. *Neurology,* 34, 939–944.

McQuade, C. E. (1981). Aging and the bereaved parent. *Widowed Persons Service—Post Conference Report.* Washington, DC: Widowed Persons Service.

Mendels, J. (1970). *Concepts of depression.* New York: John Wiley.

Merrill, T. (1974). *Discussion topics for oldsters in nursing homes.* Springfield, IL: Charles C Thomas.

Metropolitan Life Insurance Company. (1977). *Statistical Bulletin: January,* 58.

Meyerhoff, B. (1978). *Number our days.* New York: Simon & Schuster.

Mitchell, J. B. (1982). Physician visits to nursing homes. *Gerontologist,* 22, 45–48.

Moberg, D. D. (1968). Religiosity in old age. In B. L. Neugarten (Ed.) *Middle age and aging* (pp. 497–508). Chicago: University of Chicago Press.

Monk, A. (1975). Retirement—A dirty word, a depressing time. *Psychology Today,* 9, 58–63.

Monk, A. (1979). Family supports in old age. *Social Work, 24,* 533–538.

Monk, A. & Kaye, L. W. (1982). The ombudsman volunteer in the nursing home: Differential role perception of patient representations for the institutionalized aged. *Gerontologist,* 22, 194–199.

Moon, M. (1983). The role of the family in the economic well-being of the elderly. *Gerontologist,* 23, 45–50.

Morris, R., & Binstock, R. H. (1966). *Feasible planning for social change,* New York: Columbia University Press.

Mortimer, E. (1982). *Working with the elderly,* London: Heinemann Educational Books.

Moss, F. E., & Halamandaris, V. J. (1977). *Too old, too sick, too bad.* Germantown, MD: Aspen Systems Corp.

Murray, C. D., & Glassberg, D. E. (1975). Long-term health care for the elderly: The challenge of the next decade. *The Albany Law Review,* 39, 617–659.

National Center for Health Statistics. (1983). Advance Report, 1980. Monthly Vital Statistics Report, 32, 4. Hyattsville, MD: (PHS) 83–1120.

National Council on Aging (1981). *Report on the mini-conference on senior centers,* Washington, DC: N.C.O.A.

National Institute of Mental Health (1976). *Aged patients in long-term care facilities: A staff manual*. Rockville, MD: (ADM) 76–154.

National Institute of Mental Health (1979). Maintenance of family ties of long-term care patients. Rockville, MD (ADM) 79–400.

Neugarten, B. L. (1974). Age groups in American society and the rise of the young-old. *The Annals, 415*, 187–198.

Neugarten, B. L. (1977). Personality and aging. In J. E. Birren & K. W. Schaie (Eds.), *Handbook of the psychology of aging*. New York: Van Nostrand Reinhold.

Nev, A. (1976). Joint J.A.S.A./J.A.C.Y. Federation: Safety outreach program. *J.A.S.A. Brookdale News, 8*, 1–3.

Newsline. (1979). Hospice movement: A growing trend. *Geriatrics, 34*, 12.

New York Business Group on Health. (1982). Home health care provides a low cost alternative to acute hospital stay. *The New York Business Group on Health Newsletter*, 2, 1–8.

New York State. (1980). *Health systems agency plan: 1980–1985*. Albany, NY: New York State Health Systems Agency.

Ohnsorg, D. W. (1981). Burgeoning day care movement prolongs independent living. *Perspective on Aging, 10*, 18–20.

O'Meara, J. R. (1977). *Retirement: Reward or rejection*. New York: The Conference Board.

Oyer, H., & Oyer, J. (1979). Social consequences of hearing loss for the elderly. *Allied health and behavioral sciences*, 2, 101–109.

Packwood, B. (1981). Long-term care: Costs, financing and alternative services public and private sector policy options. In *National Journal Issues Book: The Future of Health Care—Current Policies and Long-term Consequences*. pp. 53–57.

Palmore, E. (1979). Predictors of successful aging. *Gerontologist, 19*, 427–431.

Park, C. C., & Shapiro, L. N. (1976). *You are not alone*. Boston: Little, Brown.

Parker, C., & Somers, C. (1983). Reality orientation on a geropsychiatric unit. *Geriatric Nursing*, 163–165.

Parnicky, J. J., Anderson, D. L., Nakoa, C. M. L. S., & Thomas, W. T. (1961). A study of the effectiveness of referral. *Social Casework, 42*, 494–501.

Peterson, J. A. (1979). *On being alone*. Washington, DC: National Retired Teachers Association.

Poister, T. H. (1978). *Public program analysis: Applied research methods*. Baltimore: University Park Press.

Rakowski, W., & Hickey, T. (1981). Geriatric patients and family resource persons: Examining congruence of health beliefs and temporal perspective. Ann Arbor, MI: The University of Michigan.

Rathbone-McCuan, E., & Hashimi, J. (1982). *Isolated elders: Health and social interventions*. Rockville, MD: Aspen Systems.

Reiff, T. R. (1980). When a patient is admitted to a nursing home. *Geriatrics, 35*, 87–94.

Reisberg, B. (1983). *Alzheimer's disease: The standard reference*. New York: Free Press.

Riegel, K. F., & Riegel, R. M. (1972). Development, drop and death. *Developmental Psychology*, 2, 306–319.

Riley, M., & Foner, A. (Eds.) (1968). *Aging and society (Vol. 1): An inventory of research findings*. New York: Russel Sage Foundation.

Robinson, B. (1983). Characteristics of the housebound elderly. Paper presented at the 36th Annual Meeting of the Gerontological Society of America. San Francisco.
Rose, A. M. (1965). The subculture of aging. In A. M. Rose & W. Peterson (Eds.), *Older people and their social world*. Philadelphia, PA: F. A. Davis.
Rosen, G. (1968). *Madness in society*. New York: Harper Torchbooks.
Rowland, K. F. (1977). Environmental events predicting death for the elderly. *Psychological Bulletin, 84*, 349–372.
Rowles, G. D. (1981). The surveillance zone as meaningful space for the aged. *Gerontologist, 21*, 304–311.
Russel, E. W. (1981). The pathology and clinical examination of memory. In S. B. Filskov & T. J. Boll (Eds.), *Handbook of clinical neuropsychology* (pp. 287–319). New York: Wiley-Interscience.
Sahlins, M. D. (1965). On the sociology of primitive exchange. In M. Bantom (Ed.), *The relevance of models for social anthropology* (pp. 220–248). London: Travistock.
Sainsbury, P. (1955). *Suicide in London: An ecological study*. London: Chapman & Hall.
Salamon, M. J. (1979). Biases in treating depression. *Geriatrics, 34*, 79–84.
Salamon, M. J. (1981). Are senior centers really for seniors? *New England Journal of Human Services, 3*, 26–30.
Salamon, M. J. (1982, April). *Approaching an objective continuum for the assessment of functionality*. Paper presented at the 3rd Annual Meeting of the Northeastern Gerontological Society, Albany, NY.
Salamon, M. J. (1983a). *Demographic factors, health care environment and life satisfaction in the elderly*. Unpublished doctoral dissertation, Hofstra University.
Salamon, M. J. (1983b). Tensions in the family. *Clinical Gerontologist, 2*, 67–69.
Salamon, M. J. (1984a). Aphasia, singing and rapport. *Clinical Gerontologist, 3*, 40–41.
Salamon, M. J. (1984b). *Chronological age and fantasy age in the elderly*. Unpublished manuscript.
Salamon, M. J. (1984c, April). *Functional assessment: A psychometric evaluation of the DMS 1*. Paper presented at the 5th Annual Meeting of the Northeastern Gerontological Society, Philadelphia.
Salamon, M. J. (1985a). A clinical application for life satisfaction. *Clinical Gerontologist, 4*, 60–62.
Salamon, M. J. (1985b). *Activities, Adaptation and Aging, 7*, 111–112.
Salamon, M. J., Charytan, P. & McQuade, C. E. (1982). Preventive health care for the elderly: A model for senior centers. *Journal of Jewish Communal Service. 58*, 115–122.
Salamon, M. J., Charytan, P., McQuade, C. E., & Friedman, D. B. (1982, March). *Senior centers and health prevention*. Paper presented at the 32nd Annual Conference of the National Council on Aging, Washington, DC.
Salamon, M. J., & Grodin, S. (1982). *Salesmanship in human services*. Paper presented at the 3rd Annual Meeting of the Northeastern Gerontological Society, Albany, NY.
Salamon, M. J., & Nichol, A. (1982). Rx for recreation. *Aging, 333/334*, 18–22.
Salamon, M. J., & Trubin, P. (1983). Difficulties in senior center life: Group behaviors. *Clinical Gerontologist, 2*, 29–39.
Schlossberg, N. K., & Entine, A. D. (1978). *Counseling adults*. Monterey, CA: Brooks/Cole.

Schmale, A. H. (1972). Giving up as a final common pathway to changes in health. *Advances in Psychosomatic Medicine*, 8, 641–650.

Schoenberg, B., Gerber, I., Wiener, A., Kutscher, A. H., Peretz, D., & Carr, A. C. (Eds.). (1975). *Bereavement: Its psychosocial aspects*. New York: Columbia University Press.

Scriven, M. (1972). Methodology of evaluation. In C. H. Weiss (Ed.), *Evaluating action programs: Readings in social action and education* (pp. 167–191). Boston, MA: Allyn & Bacon.

Shanas, E. (1971). Measuring the home health needs of the aged in five countries. *Journal of Gerontology*, 26, 68–75.

Shanas, E. (1979). Social myth as hypothesis: The case of the family relations of older people. *Gerontologist*, 19, 3–9.

Shuval, J. T., Antonovsky, A., & Davies, A. M. (1970). *Social functions of medical practice*. San Francisco, CA: Jossey Bass.

Silverstone, B. (1974). *Establishing resident councils*. New York: Federation of Protestant Welfare Agencies.

Silverstone, B., & Hyman, H. E. (1976). *You and your aging parent*. New York: Pantheon Books.

Simmons, L. W. (1945). *The role of the aged in primitive society*. New Haven, CT: Yale University Press.

Smith, D. W., Hanley-Germain, C. F., & Gips, C. D. (1971). *Care of the adult patient*. Philadelphia, PA: J. B. Lippincott.

Social Security Administration. (1982, September). Office of the Actuary Newsletter.

Somers, A. R., & Somers, H. M. (1977). *Health and health care: Policies in perspective*. Germantown, MA: Aspen Systems Corp.

Spiller, B. (1980). *The home visiting handbook of home activities programs*. New York: Associated YM-YWHA's of Greater New York.

Spreitzer, E., & Snyder, E. (1974). Correlates of life satisfaction among the aged. *Journal of Gerontology*, 29, 454–458.

Stabler, N. (1981). The use of groups in day centers for older adults. *Social Work with Groups*, 4, 49–58.

Steer, R. A., & Boyer, W. P. (1975). Milieu therapy with psychiatrically-medically infirm patients. *Gerontologist*, 15, 138–141.

Steinhauer, M. B. (1982). Geriatric foster care: A prototype and implementation issues. *Gerontologist*, 22, 293–300.

Storandt, M. (1983). *Counseling and therapy with older adults*. Boston, MA: Little, Brown.

Strain, J. J. (1981). Agism in the medical profession. *Geriatrics*, 36, 158–163.

Streib, G. F. (1971). *Retirement role and activities* (Background paper for the 1971 White House Conference on Aging). Washington, DC: U.S. Department of Health, Education and Welfare; Administration on Aging.

Sudman, S. (1976). *Applied sampling*. New York: Academic Press.

Sweetster, D. (1964). Mother–daughter ties between generations in industrial settings. *Family Process*, 33, 326–346.

Szasz, T. S. (1970). *The manufacture of madness*. New York: Dell.

Terris, B. J. (1977). Legal services for the elderly. In J. R. Barry & C. R. Wingrove (Eds.), *Let's learn about aging* (pp. 202–228). Cambridge, MA: Schenkman Publishers.

Terry, R. (1983). Current research. *The Martin Steinberg Symposium on Alzheimer's disease and related disorders*. Riverdale, NY: The Hebrew Home for the Aged at Riverdale.

Thompson, M. C. (1980). *Health policy: The legislative agenda*. Washington, DC, Congressional Quarterly Inc.

Toseland, R., & Sykes, J. (1977). Senior citizen center participation and other correlates of life satisfaction. *Gerontologist, 17*, 235–241.

United States Bureau of the Census. (1980). *Annual housing survey*. Unpublished.

United States Bureau of the Census. (1982a). Decennial census of the population, 1900–1980, and projections, 1982–2050. *Current Population Reports*, Series P-25. No. 922.

United States Bureau of the Census. (1982b). Money income and poverty status of families and persons in the United States. *Current Population Reports*, Series P-60, No. 140.

United States Department of Commerce. (1980). *Statistical abstract of the United States—1979*. Washington, DC: U.S. Bureau of the Census.

United States Federal Register. (1973, July 31). 44(148), 45036.

United States Federal Register. (1979, October 11). 38(196), 28039–28053.

United States General Accounting Office. (1978). Home health care, cheaper than nursing homes. *Aging*, 328, 9–12.

United States General Accounting Office. (1982). *The elderly remain in need of mental health services* (Report No. GAO/HRD 82-112). Gaithersburg, MD: Author.

United States Senate Select Committee on Aging. (1981). *Families: Aging and changing*. Washington, DC: U.S. Government Printing Office.

United States Senate Special Committee on Aging, Subcommittee on Long-Term Care. (1974–1976). *Nursing home care in the United States: Failure in public policy*. Washington, DC: U.S. Senate.

United States Senate Special Committee on Aging, Subcommittee on Long-Term Care. (1975). *Nursing home care in the united states: Failures in public policy. Supporting paper no. 3: Doctors in nursing homes—The shunned responsibility*. Washington, DC: U.S. Senate.

United States Senate Special Committee on Aging. (1982). *Developments in aging*. (Vol. 1). Washington, DC: U.S. Senate.

United States Senate Special Committee on Aging, (1985). *Aging America: Trends and Projections*, Washington, DC: U.S. Senate.

Vaillant, G. E. (1977). *Adaptation to life*. Boston: Little, Brown.

Verbrugge, L. M. (1983). Women and men: Mortality and health of older people. In N. M. Riley, B. B. Hess, & K. Bond (Eds.), *Aging in society: Selected reviews of recent research*. Hillsdale, NJ: Lawrence Erlbaum Associates.

Vladeck, B. C. (1980). *Unloving care: The nursing home tragedy*. New York: Basic Books.

Ward, R. A. (1979). The meaning of voluntary association participation to older people. *Journal of Gerontology, 34*, 438–445.

Warheite, G., Bell, R. A., & Schwab, J. J. (1974). *Planning for change: Needs assessment approach*. Washington, DC: The National Institute of Mental Health.

Watts, W. J. (1980). Psychological aspects of acquired deafness in old people. *Hearing, 35*, 262–264.

Weiner, M. B., Brok, A. J., & Snadowsky, A. M. (1978). *Working with the aged: Practical approaches in the institution and community*. Englewood Cliffs, NJ: Prentice-Hall.

Weiss, C. H. (1975). Evaluation research in the political context. In E. L. Streuning & M. Guttentag (Eds.), *Handbook of evaluation research* (vol. 1) (pp. 13–26). Beverly Hills, CA: Sage.

Wentowski, G. J. (1981). Reciprocity and the coping strategies of older people: Cultural dimensions of network building. *Gerontologist, 21*, 600–609.

White House Conference on Aging. (1981). *Summary reports of the committee chairmen, December 3, 1981*. Washington, DC: U.S.G.P.O.

Willemain, T. R., & Mark, R. B. (1980). The distribution of intervals between visits as a basis for assessing and regulating physician services in nursing homes. *Medical Care, 18*, 427–441.

Wilson, E. D., Fisher, K. H., & Fugua, M. E. (1975). *Principles of nutrition*. New York: John Wiley.

Index

Index